Our Unsystematic
Health Care System

Our Unsystematic Health Care System

Third Edition

Grace Budrys

ROWMAN & LITTLEFIELD PUBLISHERS, INC.
Lanham • Boulder • New York • Toronto • Plymouth, UK

Published by Rowman & Littlefield Publishers, Inc.
A wholly owned subsidiary of The Rowman & Littlefield Publishing Group, Inc.
4501 Forbes Boulevard, Suite 200, Lanham, Maryland 20706
http://www.rowmanlittlefield.com

Estover Road, Plymouth PL6 7PY, United Kingdom

British Library Cataloguing in Publication Information Available

Library of Congress Cataloging-in-Publication Data

Budrys, Grace, 1943–
  Our unsystematic health care system / Grace Budrys. — 3rd ed.
    p. ; cm.
  Includes bibliographical references and index.
  Summary: "This book presents readers with a comprehensive overview of the U.S.
health care delivery system. The third edition has been significantly revised throughout to
explain the Patient Protection and Health Care Affordability Act as it unfolds. Other key
updates include more detailed discussions of health insurance, expanded information on
health systems in other countries, and new case studies"—Provided by publisher.
  ISBN 978-1-4422-1068-4 (cloth : alk. paper) — ISBN 978-1-4422-1069-1 (pbk. : alk.
paper) — ISBN 978-1-4422-1070-7 (electronic)
  I. Title.
  [DNLM: 1. Delivery of Health Care—United States. 2. Health Care Reform—United
States. 3. Health Policy—United States.

W 84 AA1]
  362.10973—dc23   2011036133

♾™ The paper used in this publication meets the minimum requirements of
American National Standard for Information Sciences—Permanence of Paper
for Printed Library Materials, ANSI/NISO Z39.48-1992.

Printed in the United States of America

Contents

Preface   vii

1   An Interdisciplinary Overview of the Health Care System   1

2   Health Care Reform—Why Now?   15

3   Hospitals and Other Health Care Organizations   29

4   Health Care Occupations   47

5   Private Health Insurance   69

6   Public Health Insurance   89

7   Opinions on the Health Care Reform Act   105

8   The Health Care Systems in Other Countries   121

9   Health Care Policy—Making the Right Choices   141

Notes   153

Index   163

About the Author   167

Preface

In the two previous editions of this book, I focused on events that helped shape our health care system and on earlier reform proposals that did not succeed. This edition is dedicated to the daunting task of working through the changes brought about by passage of the Patient Protection and Health Care Affordability Act in March of 2010. What is special about this discussion is that this legislation is not something that everyone in the country is happy about, meaning that efforts to repeal the law or parts of the law are actively being pursued. In other words, it is not at all clear what the organizational structures envisioned by the law will look like as all the forces in favor and those that are opposed battle it out. New developments seem to appear overnight; some function as trial balloons that vanish in a few days while others continue to evolve.

I want to make clear that the picture of the health care system I am presenting is the way it looks in June of 2011. I am certain that this picture will change. However, I cannot predict how it will change. You will have to assume responsibility for following up.

This edition differs from the first two editions in a number of other ways as well. In the first two editions, I relied on sociological theory to provide the foundation for understanding the health care system as a social institution. While I still think that it is a very valuable perspective, I find that the insights offered by a number of other disciplines, particularly political science and economics, help to lay out a far more comprehensive assessment of how this institution operates. Moreover, there has been far more conceptual integration across disciplines than has been true in the past. This phenomenon is providing a far richer depiction of the range of elements that are influencing the course of health system development. Besides, it is interesting to me to discover the extent to which this new interdisciplinary approach relies on sociological concepts that were so central to the discussion I presented in the chapter on sociological perspectives in the first two editions. The second chapter outlines the reasons behind the evolution of the interdisciplinary approach.

Another change in this edition is the amount of space allotted to health insurance. Private health insurance plans and public health insurance programs are covered in separate chapters. This change is attributable to the fact that the health reform legislation devotes most attention to revising our health insurance arrangements. The discussion presented in the first chapter attends to the question of what was happening in this country that made health reform possible at this time. I have also expanded the chapter on health systems in other countries to include more countries because policy makers in the United States have referred to arrangements in other countries to a greater extent in the recent past than they were doing some years ago. Finally, rather than summarizing it all in the final chapter, I present a handful of case studies to show that everywhere we turn in deciding how the health system should operate presents dilemmas. The chapter concludes our discussion by considering the role that factors, other than the health care system, might play in explaining why Americans do not enjoy better health and longer life expectancy.

Many people have helped me get to this point. I would like start by thanking the individuals, whose names I do not know, who agreed to review what I proposed to do in this version of the book and gave it a positive reaction. And, of course, I thank all those who have chosen to adopt earlier editions of the book, giving me the courage to develop a revised version. I would also like to acknowledge the input of colleagues who listened to me expound on the issues that I address in the book and were willing to share their insights with me. Colleagues who took on the task of reading early drafts of selected sections deserve special thanks, Fernando DeMaio in particular. I am very pleased to recognize the important role that a few other people have played. Sarah Stanton, the acquisitions editor at Rowman & Littlefield Publishers, has not only given me encouragement and support but specific, practical advice. I feel very fortunate to know that she is overseeing this endeavor. Melissa McNitt, who is editing the manuscript, is remarkable. I have never had anyone do such a careful job of editing. It has made me confident that my errors have been caught. Finally, Jin Yu, assistant to Sarah Stanton, has been quick to respond to all my inquiries and cheerful about it every time. I am really grateful to these three people for making the process of moving from my electronic scribbles to a product that I can be proud of so easy.

Finally, I would like to state how grateful I am to my husband, Dan Lortie, who listened to my endless talk about health reform, gave me feedback on early and late chapters of the manuscript, and, most importantly, was always there when I was feeling upset and overwhelmed in the face of all the fuss that health reform was producing in the public media if not the scholarly press.

• 1 •

An Interdisciplinary Overview
of the Health Care System

This book is about the U.S. health care delivery system. Its basic purpose is to explain how the health care system came to look the way it does and how it is changing in response to major health care reform legislation, the Patient Protection and Affordable Care Act, enacted in March of 2010. The law has come to be known as the Affordable Care Act, or ACA. As you may already know, and as poll findings we will be discussing later will clearly confirm, a very large number of people in this country do not understand how the health care system works and admit to being thoroughly confused about the changes the health care reform is bringing. Then there are those who are sure they know what is happening and are angry about it, mainly those who think that the new legislation means that the government is trying to take over the health care system. Others, of course, think the government is doing too little, in fact cutting back on its commitment to provide health care coverage for many who depend on the government for the health care they are receiving. Have you heard about all those elderly people showing up at events in the spring of 2011 where their political representatives were scheduled to appear? All those elderly folks have been very vocal in expressing their dissatisfaction about proposals to cut Medicare funding. In short, Americans can agree that much is wrong with the U.S. health care system; yet they are in complete disagreement about how to fix what is wrong with it.

We will be encountering a lot of complicated information in this book, buried in a lot of unfamiliar terms, and loaded down with statistics and trend data. Your job is to look at the big picture. Because we are coming to this discussion just as the health care system is about to undergo tremendous changes, expect to find a steady stream of new information about the implications of the law being tossed around by people representing all kinds of interests in the media while you read this book. You are sure to hear how much difficulty particular parties are having in dealing with the requirements specified by the new law and what they are doing about that. That may sound like a lot of inexplicable commotion to you. For my part, I think this is an exciting time to be looking at our health system or, as I see it, our "unsystematic" system. I will try to make our journey into this huge quagmire as stimulating as I can, which means that I am not always as reverent about it as I might be. My objective is to keep you interested and alert.

The discussion focuses on developments over the last six decades or so that have shaped the current health care system. We will be looking at the circumstances that gave rise to the new structures and programs that were established and how well they turned out. We will also try to identify the factors that led to the most recent wave of reforms. We devote attention to what the health care system looked like before reform was enacted in order to comprehend what benefits the ACA is expected to achieve. One thing of which we can be certain is that the implementation process, however smooth or troublesome it turns out to be, will have a profound effect on the extent to which the programs and entities created by the ACA actually achieve what the reform law intends. Quite a few health care system participants have made it clear they will resist making the changes required by the law. Thus, what the law looks like on paper may not have much in common with what you see taking shape as you read this account.

In short, our unsystematic system promises to become even more unsystematic before things settle down, and you are in a position to witness that process as it is takes place. So with that introduction to how this venture will go, let's begin.

IS OUR SYSTEM THE BEST IN THE
WORLD OR SERIOUSLY FLAWED?

For years, when asked what they think of our health care system, Americans have been registering a long list of things they don't like about it. However, those same Americans have also been likely to conclude that, in spite of all that, ours is still the best system in the world.

Consider the most basic indicators. First, Americans don't live as long as people in many other developed and developing countries. According to the National Center for Health Statistics, in 2007 (the last year for which data are available at this writing), males in twenty-three of the thirty most economically advanced countries had a longer life expectancy than males in this country and females in twenty-four of the thirty most economically advanced countries had a longer life expectancy than females in this country.[1] Twenty-eight of those thirty countries also had a lower rate of infant mortality than we did in 2006.[2] Infant mortality (death of babies under one year of age) is considered the most sensitive measure of the health of a society because babies are the most vulnerable. Our infant death rate that year was 6.7 babies out of a 1,000; in Iceland the rate was 1.4; in Luxembourg, it was 2.5; in Japan it was 2.6 and in Sweden 2.8. And for this, we pay a whole lot more than anyone else in the world.

So what makes our system the "best"? It's our technology, right? We have the best medical technology in the world, and we have lots of it. So why is it that all that technology isn't doing much for our life expectancy? Because people smoke, drink, eat the wrong things, don't exercise? Anyone who travels to other countries can't help but notice that people in many other countries smoke a lot more, drink more, eat rich foods, don't exercise, and still live a lot longer.

Maybe it's because there is something wrong with the way our health care system is organized. When pressed, the defenders of our health care system are willing to acknowledge that not everyone benefits from our technology. Not because it isn't there, they point out, but because people aren't taking advantage of what is readily available. The defenders generally go on to say that highly sophisticated health care services and technology are available to everyone. Public hospitals have it and will provide it for free to those who can't pay for it. If people don't use it, you can't do anything to make them use it.

Most people involved in studying the health care delivery system would say that it is more accurate that some people are *prevented* from benefiting from the advantages provided by high-quality medical care including the latest technology. The same people would also say that we should be trying to do something about that. In my view it is the people not closely involved in studying the health care system and its impact on people in this country who are arguing that we are doing enough, and, in fact, may be doing too much. We return to these observations in almost all of the remaining chapters of the book.

When all else fails to convince skeptics, like me, that this is the best system in the world, people tend to throw down the final piece of evidence they are certain will be convincing, as if it was the missing ace in the royal flush they hold in their hands and a huge bet is riding on it. They point out that people from other countries come here to get health care because they know that it is the best system in the world. I have an answer for that, but I think I will hold off telling you why I think that happens until chapter seven, when we consider what people think of the new law; my answer is likely to produce frustration at this point.

We might want to look more closely at a couple of assumptions in the statements about health care services in general and technology more specifically. First, let's consider the assumption that the level of technology in other countries is not as advanced. That is simply not true in the case of the major industrialized European countries, Japan, and a couple of the other economically advanced countries in Southeast Asia. They have the same kind of technology, and in some cases a lot more of it. We return to this issue in chapter eight, which discusses health care systems in other countries. You may be even more surprised to find that we are not the most technologically creative. Finland turns out to have the most patents for new technology of all sorts of any country, certainly far more than we do.[3]

The second built-in assumption is that more technology is always better. After all you can get a CT scan on every corner in this country and that's great—right? In actuality, health care policy makers in the United States and other countries discovered some time ago that the doctors and technicians who perform various "high-tech" procedures and tests must do a certain number of them on a regular basis to maintain a high level of proficiency. Having many machines may mean that the people operating them, or, worse yet, interpreting the results, are not experienced enough to do a good job—to recognize aberrations, to interpret the significance of subtle differences, and so on. Not only is that hard to hear, but it strikes at the heart of the claim that lots of technology is good.

Where does that leave us in evaluating our health care system? How should we interpret the fact that one minute Americans are saying that our health care system is seriously flawed and the next that it is the best health care system in the world? It helps to understand that different people say these things and are registering different kinds of complaints about how things are working. However, having a better understanding of what people mean when they say these things is important if we are going to fix those aspects that are upsetting people so that a greater number of Americans can say they are satisfied.

Are you beginning to wonder why we are devoting this much attention to what people say about our health care system—other than to satisfy idle curiosity? Public attitude plays a major role in shaping policy decisions and votes in Congress. In other words, public opinion surveys matter a lot and for that reason must be carefully designed and conducted. It helps to find that a large proportion of the public is either strongly in favor or strongly opposed to particular proposals. This suggests that we should be looking at the results of polls carried out by well-established survey research organizations and analyzed by respected scholars. We will do some of that in the following chapter where what we have just suggested will be confirmed, namely, that Americans may agree that there is a lot wrong with our health care arrangements, but are highly divided about what they want to be changed. We return to the matter of public opinion again in chapter seven.

HEALTH SYSTEM GOALS

The discussion above should not be taken to mean that there is no agreement on what we want our health care system to accomplish. Health care policy makers and most other interested observers agree on the importance of the three guiding principles that have shaped the structure of our health care arrangements for well over half a century. They are not formally documented and written down anywhere for good reason: we don't have an organized "system." Nevertheless, the three health system goals that it is fair to say have been behind many of the reform efforts that we discuss in this book are: 1) *quality*, 2) *access*, and 3) *cost containment*.

Great goals, right? Unfortunately, that is where things get a little tricky. In part, because some interested parties may believe that one of these goals merits far more attention than the other two. Making things much more complicated is the fact that these objectives are impossible to define concretely and even more difficult to measure. What does "quality" mean? Who should define it?—doctors, patients, or some group of experts authorized (by whom?) to monitor quality? How much "access"? Does access mean that patients are entitled to have all the health care services they want? Or, that they can pay for? That someone else, say politicians, decides what they need? How do we measure "cost containment"? Do we want costs to drop or just not go up so fast? Are we prepared to cut anything? Those are exactly the kinds of questions we will be addressing in the chapters that follow.

The lack of consensus regarding the definition of access, quality, and cost containment has not stopped researchers from attempting to define and measure these things. What is special about this field of study is that scholars from multiple disciplines have been attracted to the field and have been struggling with these challenges. They may focus on somewhat different aspects of the health care system, but they all focus on topics that are related in some way to the three goals we have just identified.

Accordingly, we will be looking at the information that scholars from different disciplines present us with, which you should have no trouble understanding even though you probably do not have a strong background in the theoretical underpinnings of all of the different disciplines involved. Hardly anyone does. I will not go so far as to suggest that I expect you to remember all the facts you come across, only that I expect that you will understand what you read while you are reading it and have full comprehension of the main features of the country's health care delivery system when you finish reading this book.

ANALYTICAL PERSPECTIVES

The study of the full range of health care issues has evolved into an interdisciplinary enterprise over the last few decades. Indeed, it has become an international, interdisciplinary enterprise. A couple of decades ago, data from the United Kingdom indicating that socioeconomic status was related to the rate at which life expectancy was increasing captured the attention of everyone in this field of study.[4] It led to an enormous amount of international effort aimed at identifying the factors related to socioeconomic status that would explain these trends. The fact that everyone in the country has government-sponsored health insurance made the task of finding out what was responsible for the trends all the more challenging because it clearly eliminated the most obvious answer, that is, access to health care services. That left researchers with questions such as: Is it that those with more money are making better food choices? Is it that better education leads to better understanding of a whole range of lifestyle choices that might make a difference? Researchers from various other countries began investigating whether life expectancy followed the same pattern in their countries. They discovered that the pattern was more prevalent in some countries than in others. A recent review of the literature that focuses on this question identifies some very clear patterns to which we will return briefly in the last chapter. This field of study is known as population health research.

It is easy to understand why the field became both interdisciplinary and international once you consider the impact of the Internet. So much more information is accessible now than was true even a couple of decades ago. Information and interpretation of that information is being disseminated both more widely and more quickly. While this was happening, some other very important developments were taking shape that would add even more information and an even wider scope of interpretation.

New nonprofit foundations focusing on health care and other related social trends started to appear and older, well-established foundations began to expand. Their intent was to speak to the educated public and to provide policy makers with relevant facts about issues on which the foundations wanted to take a stand. Persons heading up the foundations were interested in taking a position on social issues backed up with solid data grounded in scientific research methods. They were particularly interested in presenting the data analyses and resulting policy statements in language that the public would understand. In order to fulfill these objectives, the foundations proceeded to hire researchers and analysts with various disciplinary backgrounds who had experience working on health care issues.

In the meantime, researchers working for government agencies began publishing research results of the reports they were working on as soon as the data became available. While data collected by the government has always been accessible to anyone who was interested, government reports are often lengthy and difficult to slog through. The fact that researchers on the inside of the data collection process were willing to present analyses of portions of those reports in a timely manner was a welcome development. A number of new interdisciplinary academic journals leaning toward policy research formed to make publication of all this new material possible.

Research being published by people in foundations and government agencies differed from work published by scholars in academic settings from which most of these researchers had come. In academia people from different disciplines had, and generally continue to have, no reason to work across disciplinary lines. In these new settings, highly trained researchers were suddenly forced to communicate with people who did not share the same disciplinary background and to do so in a way that did not depend on the venerated academic tradition that requires discussion to be grounded in theory, typically theory exclusive to a particular discipline. The upshot is that researchers trained in traditional academic disciplines who developed an interest in health care issues have become more closely connected to interdisciplinary fields such as health services research or population health research—and ready to remove any barriers that would make it hard to share information and insights.

Consequently, people trained as physicians, public health researchers, sociologists, economists, and political scientists, to name a few of the disciplinary backgrounds involved, are talking to each other and reading each other's work. That led to the discovery that concepts developed by colleagues' disciplines can be adopted without the need to understand the original contribution made by highly revered forefathers in those disciplines. The problems researchers from different disciplines choose to address continue to reflect the interests that caused them to enter into a particular program of study. What has changed is that scholars now reference each other's work across disciplines and use a wide range of shared concepts.

The kinds of questions that researchers have been addressing are far broader than they were when researchers from each discipline restricted themselves to variables and frameworks traditionally used by researchers in their respective disciplines in the past. Doctors traditionally looked at physical health indicators and disease symptoms exhibited by small numbers of people, that is, their patients. Many are now looking at disease patterns across large numbers of people and trying to identify what those people have in common that might be related to the disease. Medical economists carry out cost/benefit analyses of providing services using different approaches, economic implications of the rising cost of care on various kinds of organization, hospital mergers, physician practice costs, and so on.

Political scientists look at factors influencing the government policy decisions. They explore the extent to which public opinion is being influenced through media campaigns by those who have a lot to gain and have the resources to try to sway both public opinion and congressional voting patterns.

Sociologists look at variations in behavior and health status and health outcomes using demographic characteristics; they study the impact that particular health organizations and institutions have on the distribution of health care services. They have increasingly been focusing on determining the extent to which socioeconomic inequality affects health, as have researchers from other disciplines.

A few other disciplines have a lot to say about this field: medical anthropology, public health, and epidemiology, to name just a few. However, we will be focusing on the arguments presented by economists, political scientists, and sociologists, because they have the most to say about the central issues that we will be considering here.

One of the issues that has brought researchers from multiple disciplines together is whether delivery of health care services is best handled by the public or the private sector. What is the evidence that an arrangement driven by market competition is better—because it will deliver high-quality health care services for a cheaper price since it allows customers to have more choice? Or, is an arrangement in which the government assumes responsibility better at delivering high-quality health services at a cheaper price, since it provides equal access to those services for everyone? This question has become even more pressing in recent years because certain stakeholders have put so much effort into convincing the public that the market is superior to the government in organizing the health care system. Researchers continue to pile up evidence that relying on market solutions increases costs but this does not seem to be a message that a lot of powerful stakeholders are interested in hearing. We will get into the details of these arguments and the evidence each side offers when we focus on private insurance and public insurance in chapters five and six and the closing chapters of the book.

Advocates of one perspective or the other tend to identify themselves by the labels they attach to the two primary health care system roles. What comes closer to the role you see yourself in when you seek health care services? Are you primarily a consumer or a patient? Are you getting treated by a health care provider or a person with a more specific title such as doctor, nurse, X-ray technician, and so on? Does it make any difference? Actually it does. If you see yourself as a consumer, what follows is thinking of yourself as a knowledgeable shopper who is looking for the best buy and who is in the best position to decide what treatment you will be having. If you see yourself as a patient, your role is to accept the diagnosis of the person who has the training and experience to make that assessment. In the role of patient, your basic responsibility is to follow doctor's orders in order to get well. As is obvious, talking about the consumer role is the way proponents of market solutions want us to understand how we should think about health care services.

Discussion of the beneficial role the market plays tends to lump goods and services together. As an aside, I would like to register some reservations about treating goods and services in the same way, especially goods and services in the health care sector. You can make up your mind about many goods or products *before* you buy them, including some health care products. With services, however, you have to wait until you receive the service to decide whether or not you are satisfied. Even with that distinction in mind, the idea that members of the general public can make informed decisions about products is not always correct. Unquestionably, some people have turned themselves into informed consumers by spending an enormous amount of time researching a particular health care product or service. Most people are not prepared to do that, nor are they capable of doing it.

If you can actually test a product before you buy it, then you are better able to make an informed decision. Say it's an electric wheelchair—you can actually sit in it, drive it around, fiddle with the adjustments, and so on. You can see if there is another one that is nearly as good, but far less expensive. If you are deciding whether to opt for a generic drug or a name-brand drug—you can ask around about it, read about it, weigh lower cost against concerns you might have about products that are not made by high-profile pharmaceutical companies, but you will not know how the drug affects you until you use it because not everyone reacts exactly the same way. And you would probably learn more from having a doctor evaluate its effects than relying solely on your own assessment. Then there are products that it makes no sense to shop for. Consider a heart pump. You can't exactly decide that you need one, put in the effort to find the best one, and then try to convince a doctor to put it in your chest. The doctor decides whether you need one or not, the doctor decides which one he or she thinks will work best for you, the doctor decides whether you are ready to receive it or whether you need to do something else first, like lose X number of pounds. With health services, particularly surgery, you find out whether the surgery you signed up for produced the results you wanted after the fact.

So exactly what are we to shop for in the health care market? The strongest advocates of the market approach to health care say that Americans really want to shop for, and should be able to select, the insurance plan they like best. I am not sure about that. How interested are you in shopping for a health insurance plan? Besides, many of us can't do much comparison shopping anyway because our employers decide which plans we can choose from. How about shopping for a hospital? Is that as important as selecting the doctor you want to see, which many insurance plans restrict? Yes, we can shop for some things, but shopping for health care goods and services is not like shopping for cars, electronics, and most other consumer goods.

BUILDING A SOCIAL INSTITUTION

Let's reflect on what people say and what actually exists when we talk about the health care system. We are talking about a "social institution" that is the product of human effort. It is a structure that people are continually trying to reorganize. And the process through which it was built has not been particularly neat and orderly. We also know that the process is not about to stop, because so many observers continue to say that what we have collectively created is poorly organized, convoluted, and difficult to understand, not to mention far too expensive.

Those who study social institutions have in mind the processes and structures that exist to address a particular social need, which, in this case, is the need for health care services. The term "social institution" is not to be confused with the term "institution." We may refer to particular organizations, such as the Mayo Clinic, the Harvard Medical School, the Los Angeles County Hospital, as institutions because they are so old, well known, and widely respected. When scholars use the term "social institution," however, they are referring to all the organizations with connections to that particular sector of society—in this case the health care system. Yes, that makes it somewhat confusing. But we had to find a way to refer to multiple organizations operating in connection with each other. "Social institution" is the label we came up with. I offer this term as an example of a concept that scholars coming from other disciplines have adopted in talking about the health care system.

Until recently, health care delivery arrangements have not been considered from this perspective, because they did not attract nearly as much attention as they have been attracting over the last few decades. However, the health care delivery system has much in common with other social institutions, including education, religion, family, economy, and government.

Like the other social institutions, it evolved to address a fundamental social need and was built on the same foundation as the others. Our basic cultural values, beliefs, traditions, and expectations about the behavior of others are the building blocks that serve as the foundation on which all social institutions are constructed. This explains why social institutions change from one society to another. Each society selects from its own stock of distinctive building blocks.

True, most people have little to say about what social institutions look like. However, the choices made and opinions expressed by individuals and groups across the country are ultimately responsible for the ongoing process of shaping all of our institutions. There is generally no regularly scheduled opportunity to evaluate and possibly alter how the institution operates. That is why we are devoting a fair amount of attention to public opinion surveys. The exception to this generalization is the political system. It functions with a schedule for voting on the persons and political parties who will govern for a set period of time. The thinking regarding the operations of many other social institutions, including education, family, religion, and economics, is harder to capture and document, which makes the matter of implementing society's preferences highly uncertain.

The social institution of education provides a good illustration. As I am sure you will agree, public schools receive a fair share of steady criticism, which periodically erupts into more aggressive demands for reform. There is always someone arguing that the schools are failing our children and proposing some way to remedy the situation—creating charter schools, relying more heavily on test scores to determine which schools to support and which to close down, getting rid of teachers whose students do not show improved test scores from one year to the next and so on.

Another example of the scrutiny that social institutions undergo can be seen in the growing number of commentators who have been expressing alarm about the shifting role of religion in society. They say that we should be concerned about the steady drop in membership among traditional religions and the increase among fundamentalist sects. They argue that this brings with it more conservative views, a declining level of tolerance for behaviors such groups disapprove of, and a growing demand for restricting those behaviors. The battle over how to present sex education in schools, if at all, continues to attract the attention of parents, clerics, and other assorted interested parties, gay rights groups for example. In such cases, we can also see two or three social institutions competing to establish control over the schools and schooling. Since it is not clear whose authority and preferences should come first, or if the problems they identify really require major changes, the debates and battles continue until enough people in society are either prepared to take sides or stop listening. As a matter of fact, there is reason to think that many people are listening and are concerned about the changes taking place with regard to religion in this country. The concern is that the demands being registered by certain religious adherents are dividing the country. We will return to this development in the following chapter.

THE ORGANIZATION OF THE MATERIAL TO COME

Let's start this part of the discussion with a comment on the title of the book. I will continue to refer to the "health care system," even though most people who study health care arrangements in this country, regardless of where they stand in assessing it, would say that is it inaccurate to call what we have "a system." System suggests "systematic" and orderly arrangements. Most observers would agree that what we have is far from systematic because there is so much inconsistency across policies and programs from place to place. Calling it a system simply means that the whole social institution is the object of discussion. Calling it an "unsystematic system" may sound logically inconsistent, but it is more accurate.

There is no other way to discuss what follows, except to use the language that has evolved to address health care system issues. Get ready to encounter a fairly large number of new concepts. It's not that they are difficult to understand, it's that there are so many of them, that it is difficult to remember them all. I will try to define each new concept as it becomes central to the discussion.

References present a problem as well. If I were to give credit to everyone whose ideas I rely on, half of every page would be filled with citations. Many people have done a great deal of work that has subsequently become common knowledge, and they should be given credit for moving all of us to this stage. However, that would seriously detract from the flow of the discussion. I will provide specific citations to the work of authors whose work stands out for some reason—because it is commonly referenced, it provides very specific quantitative data, or it is particularly assertive.

There are a couple of other things that I'd like to warn you about before we jump into this venture. First, as you become more involved in this discussion—and I do, of course, hope you will become very much involved—you will undoubtedly develop opinions about how you would like to see the system work. That's good! When you present your ideas to others keep in mind that your argument will be far more convincing if you can say why you are taking the position you are taking. In other words, try to refrain from sounding like you are preaching. As in: people *should* take better care of themselves, or there *should* be more health education, or the government *should* do this or that. Telling people what they should do works fine if you are in the pulpit and conveying the word of a Greater Power. If you, as a mere mortal, tell people what they should be doing, you cannot expect listeners to treat what you say nearly as seriously. In short, you will be better off developing a strong argument based on facts as opposed to admonitions.

Second, you may feel that you already know what motivates different categories of participants to take the stance they are taking. I hope that you take care in making such observations. In order to make assertions about motivations one should be able to provide some clear evidence in support of such observations. The problem is that such evidence is generally difficult to come by. We will take up this issue in the next chapter and consider a number of factors that are playing into public perceptions of the problems that are affecting society as a whole and the health sector in particular. We will place considerable emphasis on what we can substantiate, that is, we will emphasize what people say they believe, fully recognizing that to assess people's views about a particular topic accurately at any particular time, we must ask them again and again—because people change their minds.

My third point is to ask you to be cautious in using the term "socialized medicine" even though it is being tossed around in the media as if everyone is in complete agreement on what it means. If you are referring to the systems that existed in Eastern European countries formerly affiliated with the Soviet Union, then talking about socialized medicine makes sense. The concept is also correct when applied to the system that exists in the United Kingdom, although knowledgeable persons do not use that label in connection with the UK system. When people use the term in making public presentations they do so in order to argue that whatever they are objecting to is foreign and objectionable. This is an instance in which labeling is intended to serve an important function, just as is true of the effort to convince us that we are health care consumers, not patients.

To say that something is socialized means that the government not only *runs* whatever it is, but *owns* all of the "capital" involved and *employs* all of the personnel. Translating that into health care delivery system terms means the government has total control over all the resources—it owns all the buildings (e.g., hospitals, doctors' offices, clinics); hires, fires, and pays all the personnel (doctors, nurses, technicians, aides); and, administers all of it (sets the budget, determines how many people to hire, what services to provide, where the offices should be located). This accurately describes the National Health Service in the United Kingdom. Other countries have a national insurance system. That is very different.

Countries that have "national health insurance" systems do not own hospitals or offices; and, they do not pay the salaries of all health care personnel. In most cases, doctors work on a fee–for–service basis, meaning that they receive a fee for each health care service they provide to every patient. They may be paid directly by the patients who are then reimbursed by the national health insurance system or the doctor may simply bill the national health insurance system. Other health care personnel are generally salaried by hospitals or other health care organizations, which are either fully or partially funded by the government. Hospitals in this country receive most of their income from the reimbursements that come through private insurance companies. In short, health insurance, whether it is a national system or privately purchased, is nothing more than "an insurance plan." It works very much like car insurance.

In summing up this chapter, I would like to say that this book is dedicated to the proposition that developing an informed base of knowledge constitutes an essential first step in understanding the reasons behind the successes and failures of the U.S. health care system as a social institution. The chapters to follow lay the groundwork. Given that this groundwork continues to shift, it is important to understand how the prevailing arrangements work and the intent behind the alterations that are being introduced. I hope that you conclude that having a firm background will allow you to keep up with ongoing debates. The more people who can be counted among the informed and interested, the more likely we, as a society, will understand which changes are actually going to benefit us and which will not. That should also help clarify why the prospect of making particular kinds of changes seems to produce so much heated argument and rancor.

We will attempt to develop that informed base of knowledge by considering the social, political, and economic environment in which the Patient Protection and Affordable Care Act took shape in chapter two. After that, we will take on the challenge of developing a better grasp on the operations of some of the major components of the health care system. We discuss the role that hospitals play in chapter three. In chapter four, we turn to health care occupations. In chapters five and six, we discuss the way health insurance works—first private insurance and then public insurance. We will consider what people are saying about the new health care law in chapter seven, what health care systems look like in other countries in chapter eight, and finally end by discussing a number of policy proposals and issues that are currently being debated in chapter nine.

• 2 •

Health Care Reform—Why Now?

$\mathcal{I}$n this chapter we will consider a number of issues that may help to put the debate about health care reform into perspective. The first half of the chapter outlines the factors that provided the background conditions leading to health care reform in 2010. A review of these factors raises the question of why so many previous initiatives failed. Were conditions that different this time around—different than all other times that health care policy came up for debate in this country over the last century? We will reflect on that question in the second half of this chapter.

SOCIAL PROBLEMS AND THE RECESSION

There have always been a certain number of people in this country saying that we should be doing more for the underprivileged and underserved. Their message became louder as indicators of the depth of the economic downturn that the country experienced during the first decade of the twenty-first century became more apparent. We experienced what has come to be known as the Great Recession, which, according to the National Bureau of Economic Research, started in December 2007 and ended in June of 2009. The recession was longer and more severe than any recession since World War II. Many of the people who lost their jobs, their houses, and their savings did not recover and may never recover. They obviously don't think the recession ended in 2009, and they are not so sure that anyone is trying to help them. I mention this because it helps to explain what such people have to say about the direction in which this country is going.

A number of major developments have made it difficult for people to come to some consensus regarding government actions that might help the people hit hard by the recession. For example, there is the matter of the national debt. Whether the country should try to reduce the level of debt as fast as possible or take a little more time is a huge issue but one that many Americans apparently don't understand and others have strong views about, whether or not they understand the problem. From the perspective of some politicians, and some members of the public alike, attending to the national debt requires cutting back on government spending, including how much the government spends on health care. Others are opposed to the cutbacks because so many people would not be able to pay for health care.

The concern about being able to pay for health care as well as other goods and services is connected to something else that has been occurring in this country. The development that has been getting more attention over the last few years is the evidence indicating a growing disparity between the rich and the poor. According to one leading economist, Emmanuel Saez, the inequality has not been this high since 1929.[1] That gives one pause for thought, doesn't it?

Some say that something must be done to reduce the level of socioeconomic inequality, thus increasing the pace of economic recovery and helping those hit by the recession. Yet, arguing for government intervention flies in the face of what Americans are taught from an early age, namely that everyone in this country can succeed if they try. Of course, some people are succeeding at unprecedented levels. The observations made by Robert Reich, the former U.S. Secretary of Labor and now professor of public policy at the University of California, about the rate at which the income of heads of corporate enterprises has increased make this clear.

Consider executive pay. During the 1950s and 1960s, CEOs of major American companies took home about twenty-five to thirty times the wages of the typical workers. After the 1970s, the two pay scales diverged even more. In 1980, the big-company CEO took home roughly forty times the average worker's wage; by 1990, one hundred times. By 2007, just before the Great Recession, CEO pay packages had ballooned to about 350 times what the typical worker earned.[2]

The date at which this trend took off coincides with a number of other trends to which we will return in chapter seven. For now, let's focus on another development that seems to be contributing to the problem of reaching consensus about solutions to the country's problems, namely, the growing split in social values. The 150th anniversary of the Civil War in 2011 gave historians the opportunity to make some observations comparing that era to the current era. Some of those historians maintain that this country has not faced the degree of discord that we are facing now since the Civil War era. They note that religious fundamentalists opposed to social changes occurring then were responsible for divisiveness during the period leading up to the Civil War; and that it is religious fundamentalists opposed to social changes, particularly gay marriage and abortion rights, who are responsible for much of the divisiveness we are seeing now. For their part, the fundamentalists take the position that they cannot compromise on what they consider to be sin. Accordingly, they are willing to sacrifice a great deal, particularly economic benefits, to preserve principles that are central to their belief system.

The convergence of these two developments, a very high level of economic inequality and a very high level of divisiveness concerning social values, is causing schisms that are proving very difficult to overcome. It is these schisms that are reflected in the country's inability to come together to make changes in policies that govern our health system.

It is important to recognize that this state of affairs actually serves the purposes of those who have reason to want to prevent social change. The message that those who are at the top of the economic ladder want to promote is that poor people have brought their problems on themselves—because they are lazy, have bad work habits, or indulge in other forms of personal waywardness, not because of the circumstances in which they find themselves. The people who are ready to accept this explanation for poverty are just as ready to claim that the reason some people have become very rich in the recent past is due to a combination of hard work and wise investment practices, plus one other critical factor: a healthy dose of good luck. The message is that the rich have achieved something that all Americans have a good chance of achieving. In short, don't change things before I get my chance!

At the same time, the media kept reporting that so many of the people who lost their jobs during the recession were, in fact, hardworking, upstanding members of our society who were committed to keeping their homes and way of life even as they were living from paycheck to paycheck—and that these folks were now falling into poverty. While Americans may have been ready to acknowledge the truth of this observation, they were apparently not willing to think seriously about solutions to the problem and not especially interested in reflecting on how any of this was affecting the distribution of wealth. A good illustration of this stance is reflected in a survey conducted by Michael Norton and Dan Ariely in 2010.[3] The two researchers found that Americans believe that wealth is far more equally distributed than is the case. The researchers say they cannot understand why Americans are so unwilling to acknowledge reality.

Now that we have taken a closer look at the social environment that existed just prior to the passage of the health care reform law of 2010, let's look at society's response to the troubles people faced during the Great Recession and compare that to society's response to the troubles people faced during the Great Depression. The Great Depression of 1929 stands as a serious challenge to the idea that Americans will always take the position that individuals are at fault when they have financial difficulties. Americans seemed far more willing to accept the idea that good, hard-working people could find themselves in serious financial straits then, than they are now. Indeed, this insight was responsible for passage of the Social Security Act of 1935.

HOW SOCIAL SECURITY CAME TO BE AND THE FUNCTION IT SERVES NOW

We focus on the social security program in order to reflect on why it came into existence in the first place, and to understand the role social security plays now in validating eligibility for the receipt of government health care benefits among persons over sixty-five years of age.

The Social Security Act was passed in recognition of the plight of the elderly after the economic crash of 1929. Everyone understood that the elderly were far less likely to find employment in the wake of the Great Depression than were younger people. Remember, laws against age discrimination did not exist then, so people could be forcibly retired at age sixty-five. On the other hand, no evidence suggests that the elderly were clamoring for this program. They were proud Americans accustomed to solving their own problems with the help of family members. They were opposed to government assistance defined as welfare. In other words, they shared the cultural values of the society in which they were living.

Social security became acceptable to the elderly, as well as to other members of society, when it was presented as social insurance, that is, a pension which workers would earn by contributing through a payroll tax over their work lives. The payroll tax or Federal Insurance Coverage Act (FICA) tax would go into the Social Security Trust Fund and be available upon retirement to the individual at age sixty-five.

The FICA tax was designed to rise little by little. It stands at 6.2 percent as of 2011, with the employee paying 6.2 percent, and the employer paying 6.2 percent. Observers periodically raise concerns about the solvency of the trust fund. The problem on the horizon a few decades ago was the baby boom generation beginning to reach retirement age as of 2011. This would clearly produce an imbalance between the number of people contributing to the fund and the number of people receiving benefits. The question of how to address this eventuality brought a wide range of commentators into the discussion. More recently, the concern has been that the economic downturn meant that fewer people were working and contributing to the trust fund.

Observers repeatedly mention the increase in life expectancy we have achieved since 1935 in discussing the solvency of the Social Security Trust Fund. After all, life expectancy in 1935 was fifty for men and sixty-two for women. Yes, these were indeed the life expectancy figures at that time; however, it is important to understand that life expectancy is actually calculated on the basis of the total mortality rate, including infant mortality. According to the Social Security Administration, the more appropriate measure is *adult life expectancy*. When we look at that measure, we find that men who reached the age of sixty-five in 1940 could expect to live for another 12.7 years and women could expect to live another 14.7 years. The most recent projections, from 2007, show substantial gains in life expectancy at sixty-five—males who reach age sixty-five can expect to live another 17.2 years and females can expect to live another 19.9 years. So we really are living longer. However, understanding what life expectancy figures mean and how they are calculated makes the issue more complex, doesn't it?

After deliberating the implications of increasing life expectancy for the trust fund in 1983, Congress instituted a new schedule for retirement with full benefits incrementally increasing the age of eligibility from age sixty-five to age sixty-seven on a month-by-month basis. Americans have always been able to retire earlier, at age sixty-two, with reduced benefits. That has not changed.

The solvency of the trust fund was still not assured even after this adjustment. That, in turn, led Congress to ask the trustees to assess the situation once again in 2008. This time the trustees indicated that the trust fund would be running out of money by 2017. The options were to either reduce benefits or increase taxes or some mix of both. Others argued for privatization, which translates into giving people the pension they had accrued as a lump sum to be invested as they wished. Others advocated investing the trust fund in stocks, bonds, and other financial instruments, that is, in the market. The severity of the Great Recession dampened public enthusiasm for investing in the market. The topic continues to come up without a solution that the majority in Congress and the public sphere can agree on.

Medicare solvency was projected to be extended by twelve years to 2029 by the passage of the Affordable Care Act. However, the fact that the economy was not recovering as quickly as expected caused Medicare trustees to reassess the situation the following year. In the spring of 2011, the trustees announced that by their calculations Medicare would be running out of funds by 2024. The issue of Medicare solvency once again moved up to the top of the agenda among politicians committed to reducing the size and scope of government.

Curiously, the media has made little mention of the ceiling on FICA taxes in discussions about the solvency of the Social Security Trust Fund. In 2011, FICA applies to income up to $106,800. The ceiling goes up a bit each year. However, income above that rate is not taxed. Economists point out that this is a "regressive" tax. In other words, it places a bigger burden on people at lower income levels than higher income levels. And it certainly limits the amount of money that is being contributed to the trust fund.

HEALTH CARE REFORM BETWEEN 1935 AND 1965

There was some effort to incorporate health care benefits when the Social Security Act was legislated, but coming out of the Depression, the country simply could not afford it. As a matter of fact, health care reform took a backseat to other issues on the national agenda throughout the first half of the twentieth century for a long list of reasons. To begin with, medical costs were not very high and doctors were much more willing to accept token payment, a chicken or having some house repairs done, when patients could not afford to pay the fee. Hospitals adjusted their charges depending on patients' ability to pay as well. Newspapers sometimes reported the exorbitant charges a famous movie star was asked to pay for a routine procedure, going on to say how pleased the star was about it all.

Another reason why health care reform did not receive more attention during this period is that, while the effects of the Great Depression lingered on during the decade of the 1930s, the country's attention turned to the demands brought on by World War II. Everything changed with the onset of the war. War production went into high gear. As more men became engaged in war activities, women entered the work force—working in offices and in factories. They saved the money they made, in part, because consumer goods were not available since they were not being manufactured. When the war ended, Americans were eager to make up for lost time. They bought new houses in the suburbs and cars to get there. They bought new furniture and appliances for the new houses. They had babies—creating the baby boom generation. The economy was booming. Personal income increased by 37 percent between 1950 and 1956.[4]

Health care reform did come up for serious debate during the post-war period, the late 1940s, the Truman era. It is interesting to see that 82 percent of the public favored doing something to help people pay for health care and that 68 percent agreed that using social security as the basis for enacting a universal health care plan was a good idea.[5] In spite of this high level of popular support, the proposed plan did not succeed for complicated political reasons.

Health care reform did not capture the attention of the public again until the early 1960s. Interest in health care reform during this era was inspired by the observations offered by a few highly respected social critics who pointed out that not everyone in the country was enjoying the newfound post-war prosperity. While the critics presented powerful impressionistic information, there were no factual data to which anyone could refer in discussing the scope of the problem. The government was pressed into figuring out how many poor people there were and who they were. There was no standard indicator in existence at the time that would produce a count of the number of people in the country who were poor. The government first had to establish a measure to determine who was poor and who was not. The Bureau of Labor Statistics was mandated to take on the task. It turned to the Consumer Price Index (CPI), which it had been using to set wages for workers in shipbuilding yards. The CPI involved calculation of the cost of a market basket of goods that a person would need to survive—starting with food, going on to clothing, housing, transportation, medical care, and a number of other categories, like energy.

The cost of a basket of essential goods and services, which was announced for the first time in 1961, was calculated to be $2,973 for a family of four. This established the *poverty line.* Those whose income was less than that were considered poor. So how many people were found to be poor and who were these people? More than one out of every five persons, 22 percent, turned out to have an income lower than the poverty line. Of persons between the ages of twenty-five and fifty-four, 13 percent were found to be poor; but, 47 percent of those over sixty-five were poor.[6] Of those in female-headed households 50 percent were poor; and 56 percent of African Americans were poor. The fact that this took place during the Kennedy/Johnson era, when the mood of the country was considerably more sympathetic to the plight of the needy than has been true since then, explains why the findings came to be defined as a serious national problem that the government needed to address.

The social values that prevailed during that period meant that Americans were more likely to be sympathetic to the plight of all the categories of people identified as poor. A range of social programs was legislated during this period designed to address problems faced by specific categories of people. Medicaid, civil rights legislation, and funding for education and training at all levels came into existence at this time. The fact that the elderly were having difficulty paying for health care even though they were receiving social security checks captured the attention of the country. The majority of Americans, 75 percent according to surveys conducted at the time, said they favored a plan to provide medical care for seniors.[7] This led to passage of the Medicare program in 1965.

However, policy experts did not anticipate that the costs of health care would continue to increase after the two massive government-sponsored health insurance programs, Medicare and Medicaid, came into existence. They projected a decline in health care costs once the needs of the under-served were addressed. What in retrospect looks like a relatively small but steady increase in health care costs led to the next significant piece of health care legislation. The Nixon administration introduced a major health care reform in 1974 designed to encourage people to seek care early before prob-lems got more serious. Policy experts reasoned that providing preventive care and addressing health problems at an early stage when they were less costly to treat should stem the rise in health care costs. This accounts for the origins of Health Maintenance Organizations (HMOs).

While the cost of care continued to rise, in fact, at a faster rate than it had been rising until then, health care reform received little attention during the 1980s. Americans had been hearing about the number of people who did not have health insurance and could not afford to obtain health care, but it was only when Clinton entered the political arena during the late 1980s that doing something about it, that is, talking about health care reform, became a primary goal. In fact, health care reform became one of the basic elements in Clinton's political campaign. He came into office in 1990 with 66 percent of Americans saying they favored legislation creating a tax-funded national health insurance plan.[8] Pundits found many reasons to explain why the plan never made it to the proposal stage for Congress to consider.

One explanation is that corporate executives were convinced that the plan would not succeed so it made no sense to risk coming out in support of it. That would have displeased too many influential people associated with the business sector. Ironically, many companies, particularly in the auto industry, would have benefited tremendously from the passage of health care reform. It would have reduced operating costs and given manufacturers a significant pricing advantage in the international market. In short, political interests trumped economic interests.[9]

Debates about health care reform continued to attract the public's at-tention over the next two decades because health care costs continued to rise and increasing numbers of people had trouble getting health insurance. The economic downturn during the early years of the first decade of the twenty-first century exacerbated the problem because people were losing their health insurance along with their jobs. In other words, more people could not get health care services because they could not afford to pay for health care and they could not find health insurance coverage that would make health care affordable.

This is a good place to stop and see the extent to which poverty may currently be a factor in people's inability to obtain health care and other goods and services. So how many people are we talking about? How many Americans are poor at the end of the first decade of the twenty-first century? What do poverty statistics look like after all those interventions aimed at reducing poverty over the last five decades? According to the Census Bureau, as of 2009, 14.3 percent of Americans fell below the poverty line. The rates are considerably higher for some categories: 25.8 percent of African Americans and 25.3 percent of Hispanics compared to the 9.4 percent rate for whites and 12.5 percent rate for Asians.

A closer look at age and poverty suggests that we have not been attending to the emergence of a new poverty problem. The numbers have shifted from high numbers of poor elderly to high numbers of poor children. The 2009 count reveals that 20.7 of all children under age eighteen are poor. By contrast, less than 8.9 percent of persons over sixty-five fell below the poverty line, a figure that is lower than the poverty rate of those of working age between eighteen and sixty-four, 12.9 of whom are poor. So now that you have considered the face of poverty in this country—would you say that things have gotten better and that we are moving in the right direction to address poverty or would you say that we are not doing nearly enough?

FACTORS THAT EXPLAIN THE SUCCESS OF THE 2010 HEALTH CARE REFORM

The researchers who tracked the fate of proposed health care reform legislation during the periods when there was serious discussion about reform in this country—the Truman administration (late 1940s), the Kennedy/Johnson administration (mid-1960s), the Nixon administration (1974), and the Clinton administration (early 1990s) identified two factors they said were especially important in determining whether reforms were actually enacted.[10] They concluded that the level of trust in government and feelings about federal taxes were the factors that determined whether health care reform would go forward or not. They pointed out that the level of distrust in government was especially high during the Clinton era. To put this in context, they noted that trust in government had been steadily eroding since the 1950s.

What about trust in government during the Obama administration? President Obama enjoyed very high approval ratings during the first year or two of his administration, which we might think of as a measure of trust. At the same time, we also know that the forces opposed to Obama's agenda were gathering steam. Mid-term elections resulted in the appointment to Congress of a large number of persons adamantly opposed to government, government spending, and solutions to social problems grounded in government programs.

Consequently, as of 2011, the country is more highly divided than ever. That has made governing increasingly more difficult, which in turn has caused some of Obama's supporters to lose confidence and trust in his ability to achieve the legislative goals he set forth during his campaign.

As we noted at the beginning of this chapter, the economy was continuing to deteriorate during this period. Increasing numbers of people were being laid off and losing their health insurance in the process during the first couple of years of the Obama administration. In addition, the response of the business sector was to cut back on employee benefits as the cost of health insurance continued to escalate. Therefore, not just those who lost their jobs were uninsured, but those who still had jobs were now losing their coverage as well. The numbers of people who could not pay their hospital and doctor bills increased. More people went into medical bankruptcy. This was turning into a perfect storm!

The country's sense of this is reflected in the results of a June 2009 *New York Times* poll.[11] It revealed that 85 percent of the randomly selected respondents said that the health care system required fundamental reform; at the same time, 77 percent said that they were very or somewhat satisfied with their own arrangements. Interestingly, 72 percent registered support for a plan, like Medicare, that would cover everyone. The results of the poll clearly presented policy analysts with a major challenge—how do you change things without upsetting those who like their arrangements? It did show, however, that a very high proportion of people were willing to support change of some sort.

The shift in attitude exhibited by major health sector players may have played a particularly noteworthy role. Insurance companies stopped running ads accusing government of taking over people's right to choose their own health care plans; they spent a lot of money doing this during the Clinton health care reform era. They stopped saying that health care reform signaled a socialistic takeover, which is not to say that those opposed to government programs and government spending stopped invoking the specter of government takeover. The professional associations representing hospitals, doctors, and nurses, each to a different extent, began saying that the country's health care system was broken and should be fixed. They differed in how they thought it should be fixed, but they were no longer putting up a wall against health care reform proposals. In other words, influential health sector participants began to see that they could benefit from reforms that would provide more people with health care coverage.[12]

Finally, a major factor favoring passage of the ACA health care reform act is that Democrats were in control of all three government bodies involved in enacting laws in this country—the White House, the House of Representatives, and the Senate during the first two years of the Obama administration in 2009 and 2010. The Democrats were the ones proposing health care reform each time it came up for serious discussion over the last century. This is the first time in a long time that they had the leverage and political savvy to make it happen.

Researchers who reviewed fifty opinion polls conducted since 1943 (twenty-three of those conducted between 2008 and 2010), have given us a far more detailed picture of the factors that kept health care reform from being legislated until 2010. It is interesting to see what has changed and what has stayed the same. The researchers tell us that Americans have consistently registered support for health care reform, but that their support has almost always been tempered by overriding concern about the economy. Americans have consistently registered dislike for personal sacrifice; while all along they have favored reforms that would provide health insurance for the uninsured, they have not been interested in making personal sacrifice in order to pay for that. They are inconsistent now, just as they have been in the past, in saying that they like the health care arrangements they have on the one hand and saying they are worried about being able to pay for needed care on the other hand.[13]

The political split that is reflected in American attitudes about health care reform may have existed in the past. However, it has become far more apparent in the most recent polls. Unquestionably, the decline in trust in government has played an especially important role. In 1969, the first year a question about trust was asked, 69 percent of Americans said they trusted the government; in 2010, only 19 percent said they trusted the government.[14] Another disappointing finding is the extent to which Americans are unaware of the issues that health care reform aims to address.[15] Whether they are less well informed now than they have been in the past is not entirely clear, but the degree to which they are uninformed currently is very clear.

HEALTH CARE REFORM OPTIONS

Let's take a closer look to see what is special about the Affordable Care Act of 2010 and how it differs from previous reform efforts that did not succeed. According to the Institute of Medicine (IOM) previous health care reform proposals fell into one of the following categories.[16]

1. employer mandates that require employers to provide insurance for all employees and all others to be covered by public plans
2. individual mandates requiring everyone to buy their own insurance with the aid of tax credits
3. the single-payer plan

4. the incremental approach that depends on expansion of existing public programs, i.e., Medicare, Medicaid, SCHIP (State Children's Health Insurance Program) often together with government assistance to allow the uninsured to buy into these programs

For a long time, the fourth option was the only one that most Americans would support. Thus, what makes the health care reform of 2010 so extraordinary is that it succeeded in rolling three of the four alternatives into one proposal, leaving out only the third option, the single payer plan. (We discuss this alternative in more detail in chapter seven.) It is the single-payer option that has consistently produced the strongest opposition because it is so dependent on government control over health insurance arrangements rather than competition among insurance companies in the private sector to deliver on the three health system goals—access, quality, and cost containment.

According to some of the same researchers who tracked the reasons behind the success or failure of previous health proposals, the ACA succeeded because it was able to combine a liberal goal—health insurance coverage for everyone—and a conservative approach to insurance—personal responsibility for selecting a health plan of one's own choosing.[17] That allowed the individual mandate, requiring everyone to buy health insurance, to go forward. The employer mandate, which affects small employers, could be included because the government would be providing tax relief for small employers in order to ease the financial burden. The ACA succeeded because, while the law does expand government programs, the legislation relies so heavily on the private sector, that is, insurance companies, to provide health insurance coverage to more Americans.

In other words, the "definition of the situation," as was true in the case of the Social Security legislation following the Great Depression, was successfully captured in concepts acceptable to the American public. It succeeded in making the 2010 health care reform proposal acceptable to many interested parties who had been opposed to health care reform in the past.

THE MONEY WE SPEND ON HEALTH CARE

Without a doubt, the ACA will cost the country a great deal of money. Where do Americans stand on how much the reform will cost? Does the fact that so many candidates associated with the Tea Party faction of the Republican Party, which aims to cut the government budget as much as possible, have been elected to Congress and that Republicans have gained control over the House of Representatives during the interim election of 2010 mean that most

Americans are registering disapproval for how much the country is spending or will be spending on health care?

The answer is that Americans are displeased about how much they are spending "out of pocket" on their own health care. However, they do not seem to be particularly displeased about how much the country as a whole is spending nor are they interested in examining the connection between what they spend on health care and how much the country spends on health care. How much the country spends on health care is calculated as a percentage of the Gross Domestic Product (GDP). We should discuss this concept in a little more detail.

GDP is a measure of the total of goods and services bought and sold in the country. That is certainly a straightforward definition until you start thinking about what it means. It becomes more daunting if you conceptualize it as a pie chart and understand that *all* goods and services produced or purchased by anyone and everyone in the country must fit into the pie—cell phones, cars, bridges, bombs, dental care, computers, the space program, food stamps, houses, police protection, rock concerts, and on and on. The slice of this pie that goes to health care products and services has been getting bigger over the years. Throughout the decade of the 1990s it hovered around 14 percent. According to the Centers for Medicare & Medicaid Services, it stands at 17.6 percent in 2009.[18] Government projections indicate that the percentage will increase to 19.3 by 2019.[19] Is that too much, too little, about right? Although most Americans do not seem to be interested in addressing this issue, it is probably not much of an exaggeration to say that health care policy experts and other experts who focus on the economy are getting freaked out about it.

Then there is the question of how you want that percentage of GDP divided up. As of 2008, the federal government is picking up 27 percent of the health care tab; local governments are picking up 16 percent; private business is picking up 21 percent; that leaves 28 percent for private households to cover. What is it that we are all paying for and where do we want to look for ways to cut costs? The following indicates how the health care dollar is distributed.[20]

30.7 percent	Hospital care
31.3 percent	Professional services
8.7 percent	Nursing home and home health
10.0 percent	Prescription drugs
2.8 percent	Other medical products
6.8 percent	Government administration and net cost of private insurance
3.0 percent	Public health activities
1.9 percent	Research
4.9 percent	Structures and equipment

While some of the people who object to how much we spend on health care would have us believe that cutting costs is a matter of will—to just stop spending on unnecessary goods and services—even the most superficial examination of the implications reveals that it is a whole lot more complicated than that. We will continue to raise questions about the pros and cons of making cuts in almost every chapter. The challenge to keep in mind when we address questions about where to cut is that it is easy to figure out who will gain—us, the taxpayers, but who will lose is typically not nearly as clear. Another way of putting it is—what happens when we cut back on programs? Are we prepared to support cuts that will cause some people to go without care, get sicker, die sooner? After all, people's health problems will not simply disappear if we cut government programs. Or are we really talking about shifting the costs to some other party? We know from opinion surveys that individuals have consistently been opposed to having the financial burden shifted onto them. State governments have been registering even more concern about the implications of cuts in federal programs for state budgets. So who do we want to stick with paying for the country's health care costs? That does make cutting costs seem like a more challenging problem, doesn't it?

• 3 •

Hospitals and Other Health Care Organizations

_P_eople generally don't think about hospitals unless they need to go to one because of a pressing health problem. When they do go, they are naturally preoccupied with the health problem that is causing them to be there. For purposes of this discussion we will be taking a broader view of hospitals. We will look at hospitals and other health care organizations as organizational structures, who owns them, how much we are spending on hospital care, and how hospitals and related organizations are changing.

Let's consider a number of basic characteristics that distinguish hospitals from each other. The most basic difference stems from how long patients stay in the hospital. There are short-term stay, or "acute care," hospitals and there are long-term stay hospitals. The majority of hospitals in this country are short stay hospitals. Long-term stay hospitals generally provide inpatient mental health treatment and rehabilitation. Also, some "long-term care" facilities are not hospitals, but nursing homes. Unless otherwise indicated, the discussion to follow refers to short-term, acute care hospitals.

Size is another meaningful characteristic. Counting the number of hospitals tells you something, but leaves a lot unsaid about capacity, that is, what services the hospitals are capable of delivering. There are various ways to measure capacity, including the hospital's number of employees, its annual budget, its kinds of specialty units, its number of branches, and so on. The commonly agreed-on measure of size is the number of beds the hospital maintains. A hospital in a rural area might have fifty to seventy-five beds while a medical center hospital might have five hundred beds.

Another basic distinguishing criterion is hospital ownership. Who owns the hospital makes a significant difference; the extent of the difference has inspired heated debate over the past few decades. When the government reports

29

hospital statistics, it differentiates between hospitals owned by the federal government and nonfederally owned hospitals. Federally owned and funded hospitals are basically operated by the Veterans Administration for the exclusive use of veterans of the armed forces. All other hospitals fall into the nonfederal category. They are divided into three ownership categories: 1) nonprofit, 2) for-profit, and 3) state-local government.

Hospitals in the state and local government category are the easiest to recognize. They are usually named to clearly indicate that they are government-sponsored, like Boston City Hospital, Los Angeles County Hospital, or University of Illinois Hospital. The state and local government hospitals are, in the broadest sense, not-for-profit organizations. They are typically referred to as *public* hospitals (i.e., funded by the public through taxes) to distinguish them from hospitals that are largely supported by individuals and organizations in the private sector. The same labeling is used to identify the sponsorship of other organizations in the health sector and outside of it. Any organization that is supported by taxes is considered a *public* organization.

Major university-sponsored teaching hospitals usually, but not always, carry the name of the medical schools that own and operate them. Many other hospitals are loosely affiliated with medical schools, which themselves may be publicly supported or privately supported nonprofit organizations. Affiliation with a medical school allows a hospital to offer graduate medical education in the form of residency programs. Persons who have already earned a medical doctor's degree (i.e., medical residents) carry out their postgraduate, practical, on-the-job medical training there. Medical schools have more graduates than they can accommodate at the university hospital for residency training, which takes anywhere from three to five years, more if the doctor wishes to subspecialize. For this reason, university teaching hospitals must develop ties to state and local as well as "community" hospitals to provide places for medical students and residents to receive hands-on training.

The term "community" hospital has traditionally served as a catchall label for hospitals that are owned and operated for the benefit of the community (as opposed to owners and investors). They may have been established by religious orders, leading citizens aiming to create a hospital to provide for their own religious or ethnic groups, or residents of a particular geographic community. The government has recently begun to use the "community" label more broadly to refer to all acute care hospitals regardless of ownership (as you see in table 3.1).

The for-profit category includes hospitals that are privately owned and operated as profit-making enterprises. They are not always easy to distinguish from nonprofit community hospitals. Historically for-profit hospitals were owned by individuals, usually one or more doctors. As owners, they pocketed

Table 3.1. Hospitals in the United States, 1975–2008

	1975	*1995*	*2008*
All hospitals	7,156	6,291	5,815
Federal	359	299	213
Community	6797	5992	5602
Nonprofit	3,222	3,092	2,923
For-profit	780	752	982
State-local	1,778	1,350	1,105

Source: Hospitals, beds, and occupancy rates, according to type of ownership and size of hospital: United States, selected years 1975–2008. *Health, United States, 2010: With Special Feature on Death and Dying* (Hyattsville, MD: National Center for Health Statistics, 2011), table 113 (Online at http://www.cdc.gov/nchs/data/hus/2010/113.pdf).

what they earned from running the hospital; they made all the decisions on the need for improvements, both technological and cosmetic, hiring staff, and so on. They also paid taxes on any profits. This is a major distinction. The government does not tax nonprofit hospitals. Individuals no longer own for-profit hospitals. Instead corporations own them (to make things more confusing, corporations that sell stock are sometimes referred to as "publicly owned" because many people are owners by virtue of investing in the company); these corporations aim to make a profit, sell shares to stockholders and distribute profits to those who invest in the business, and pay taxes.

The Department of Health and Human Services keeps track of the number of hospitals in each category. Some changes have taken place over time. Table 3.1 indicates the changes that have taken place over the last few decades.

Recognizing that counting the number of beds is generally considered to be a more accurate measure of hospital trends, table 3.2 reports the shift in the number of hospital beds between 1975 and 2008. As you can see the

Table 3.2. Distribution of Hospital Beds, 1975–2008

	1975		*1995*		*2008*	
	Number	*%*	*Number*	*%*	*Number*	*%*
All	1,465,828	100	1,080,601	100	951,045	100
Federal	131,946	9	77,079	7	45,992	5
Nonfederal	1,333,882	91	1,003,522	93	905,053	95
Community	941,844	100	872,736	100	808,069	100
Nonprofit*	658,195	70	609,729	70	556,651	68
For-profit*	73,495	8	105,737	12	120,887	15
State-local*	210,154	22	157,270	18	130,531	16

*percentage of community hospitals

Source: See source for table 3.1.

total number of beds has been declining since 1975. However, policy makers were most interested in following distribution of beds, especially in the fact that the number of beds in for-profit hospitals has continued to increase. Before we get to that point, let's go back to the beginning of the twentieth century to see how we got to the numbers of hospitals and hospital beds shown in these tables.

A BRIEF HISTORY OF THE MODERN HOSPITAL

Before the twentieth century, people avoided a hospital stay if they had any choice about it. Hospitals were essentially charitable organizations that provided basic care and housing for indigents who had no place else to go. Exactly how many hospitals there were in this country around the turn of the century is difficult to determine. According to one of the few estimates available, as of the mid 1880s, there were only 178.[1] People did not go into a hospital willingly because everyone knew that hospitals were dangerous places. One's chances of dying once you were in the hospital were high. Middle-class people certainly would not have paid to go there. Those who could afford it were treated in their own homes or the doctor's office. Many people also sought advice and remedies from the apothecary (i.e., pharmacist) and any number of other kinds of health practitioners.

While most people would have been reluctant to go into the hospital at the beginning of the twentieth century, surgeons were beginning to find it more difficult to perform surgery outside of the hospital. They had begun to perform more new kinds of surgery than they had been able to do even a few decades before largely due to a range of technological advances. Anesthesia, which was initially developed in the 1840s, had become more effective and reliable. (Imagine what surgery was like before anesthesia! People died from the shock of being cut open even before they had a chance to develop an infection; if they survived, infection was, of course, very likely.) The value of antisepsis (a sterile surgical environment) was discovered in the 1860s and was now fully implemented. X-ray technology came into existence in the 1890s. As surgeons became more dependent on hospitals to perform surgical procedures, they also became more interested in setting standards that would improve the quality of hospital care.

Accordingly, in 1918 the American College of Surgeons began inspecting hospitals in an effort to assure the public that hospitals were well equipped and that the doctors doing surgery were well qualified. They did so by encouraging doctors to assume greater responsibility for overseeing the work of their colleagues. They were especially concerned about preventing less-qualified or unethical colleagues from performing unnecessary surgery.[2] The medical profession as a whole, led by the most accomplished surgeons, improved the quality of care provided in hospitals by having pathologists perform autopsies on the patients who died in the hospital to determine whether the diagnosis was accurate and the surgery was truly necessary, and, of course, done well. The public nature of the autopsy meant that surgeons had to be more careful about the surgeries they were performing, because all doctors affiliated with the hospital were encouraged to attend autopsies as an excellent method to discuss cases and advance medical knowledge. Having colleagues discover that the surgeon was misdiagnosing patients and performing unnecessary surgery would certainly not be good for the surgeon's reputation.

To ensure that autopsies were, in fact, being carried out and that the privileges of doctors doing inappropriate surgeries were restricted, the American College of Surgeons encouraged doctors to become active members of the medical staff organization in the hospital. In short, doctors were encouraged to establish firm control over the day-to-day work taking place in hospitals.

Administrators of hospitals were well aware of the fact that their interests were not identical to those of surgeons, or for that matter, the interests of other physicians and other hospital personnel. They began organizing themselves into an association of their own. In 1899 they established the Association of Hospital Superintendents of the United States and Canada, which became the American Hospital Association (AHA) within the next few years. Over the next decade or so the AHA came around to the view of the surgeons that raising hospital standards was important and that inspections were essential. However, the AHA did not have the resources or the power over hospitals to impose such inspections. The American College of Surgeons did have that power.

When hospitals were primarily charitable institutions, doctors contributed their services. They did so because hospitals provided them with interesting "clinical material" (i.e., interesting cases). In other words, the patients were more likely to be in an advanced stage of disease because they did not have the money to obtain treatment earlier, often because the disease prevented them from working and impoverished them. A lot of very sick people could not afford to see a doctor privately. So doctors volunteered their services in exchange for the opportunity to treat the interesting cases. As hospital care improved, middle-class patients began asking to be admitted to the hospital, indicating willingness to pay the doctor as well as the hospital for the care they would receive. Thus began a pattern that would lead to hospitals beginning to depend on paying patients for their operating funds. Surgeons were in a position to funnel their paying patients to the hospital of their choice. Hospitals were left with little alternative but to accede to the surgeons' wishes—focusing on making the improvements that surgeons demanded, such as bigger and better surgical suites, more advanced equipment, and more staff.

The American Hospital Association first approached the American College of Surgeons around 1950 to explore the possibility of setting up a cooperative inspection program. Four organizations joined together to develop hospital accreditation standards: the American Hospital Association, the American College of Surgeons, the American Medical Association, and the American College of Physicians. By 1952 they had worked out standards and established a new organization, the Joint Commission on Hospital Accreditation, to carry out the inspections. The inspections were to be voluntary; hospitals would have to request them and be charged for the costs of carrying them out. As of 1987, it became the Joint Commission on Accreditation of Healthcare Organizations (JCAHO), generally now referred to as the Joint Commission. The role of JCAHO is very obvious to everyone employed in a hospital, especially when the Joint Commission arrives for an accreditation visit.

Hospitals expanded rapidly during the first few decades of the twentieth century, until the end of the 1930s.[3] According to one of the first American Medical Association counts, there were approximately 4,300 hospitals in the country in 1928. Then the trend suddenly reversed. The drop is attributed to the Great Depression. Patients could not afford to go to a hospital, those who were taken there because it was an emergency could not pay for it, and many smaller hospitals did not survive. The hospitals that did survive could absorb such losses only because they were receiving support from especially dedicated and, in many cases, wealthy contributors. Some hospitals survived because of the support they received from religious orders or an entire ethnic community. The only other hospitals that survived the Depression were those operated by local governments.

The hospital sector changed little between the Depression and the end of World War II. Once the war ended, however, the country experienced a period of adjustment that brought with it not only peace, but a period of unprecedented prosperity and expansion into newly developing communities. With all this expansion, there was a need for new hospitals, which brought the Hill-Burton Act into existence in 1946. The federal government matched the funds raised by the community for the purpose of building a new hospital or adding on to an existing one. Consequently, established hospitals expanded and new community hospitals sprang up all across the country.

Was there really a need for so much more hospital construction or could there have been some other reason behind the urge to build and expand? Admittedly, the definition of "need" in this case has its own body of literature. For purposes of this discussion something besides objective need is involved.

Many hospitals came into existence for symbolic reasons. They stood as a major source of pride to the community whether it was an ethnic, religious, or geographical community. The Hill-Burton Act provided the perfect opportunity to act on that sense of pride. It is also true that some urban hospitals were built by people who had good reason to believe that they were not welcome in hospitals operated by other groups. Jewish doctors, for example, experienced discrimination when seeking privileges in hospitals run by others. Jewish patients felt better being treated by doctors who they felt would understand their cultural values. Similarly, Catholic hospitals offered the assurance that patients could practice their religion and that priests would be readily available to offer solace, hear confession, and offer last rites. Immigrants were concerned about being able to communicate and wanted to be able to speak their own language in the hospital. Finally, the newly established suburban communities were interested in proving that they could offer everything that the city could offer, only newer and better. (See the social construction of reality at work here? The people building hospitals were certain there was a need for all those new hospitals and new additions—perhaps not the kind of need that policy analysts might be looking for, but, as you can see, "need" is in the eyes of the beholder.) It goes without saying that poor people in poor neighborhoods could not, and did not, take advantage of the Hill-Burton funds. For this reason, new hospitals were not built in many communities that really needed them.

Aside from community pride, one other factor that played a major role in fostering hospital expansion coincidentally came into play just after World War II ended. Synthesized penicillin came into existence during the late 1940s and became widely available by 1950. (Scientists knew about the value of penicillin in its original state, that is, mold. It took a while to identify the chemical formula so it could be produced in volume and under antiseptic conditions.) The availability of penicillin had a major effect on hospital expansion because this was the first time that hospitals could control infection with certainty. Prior to that time drugs to control infection did exist, but none was as powerful as the new series of antibiotics, starting with penicillin.

MORE RECENT DEVELOPMENTS

By the middle of the twentieth century people were not only more willing to go into the hospital, they were prepared to stay there for days. However, even at that time, staying in the hospital was not a minor expense. So who paid for people to luxuriate in the hospital for days? The answer is health insurance, initially Blue Cross, later commercial insurance, and as of 1966, Medicare and Medicaid.

The enactment of Medicare and Medicaid turns out to be a huge event for the future of hospitals and health care in general in this country. The two programs guaranteed payment on behalf of those who had been least likely to be hospitalized because they could not afford it. That brought in a lot of "new business" to hospitals, causing hospitals to grow and expand to accommodate increasing demand for health care services. (If talk about the business of health care delivery makes you think that things are finally going to be orderly and efficient, you're going to like what happens over the next few decades; if talk about the health care business makes you uncomfortable, prepare yourself, this is just the beginning. Hospitals and health care organizations are about to become BIG BUSINESS.) The expenditures on hospital care went from $9 billion in 1960 to $1.2 trillion by 2008.[4]

From the perspective of hospitals, Medicare, and to a lesser extent Medicaid, would be providing a steady, and, more importantly, reliable stream of funding from this time forward. The government wanted some assurance that government funds would be going to good, as opposed to fly-by-night, hospitals. Therefore, the government decreed that Medicare funds could only go to hospitals accredited by the Joint Commission on Accreditation of Healthcare Organizations (remember this is the voluntary association created to upgrade standards). That not only gave the Joint Commission increased power, but it eliminated hospitals that could not successfully pass a review by the Joint Commission because they could not compete with hospitals that were eager to emphasize that they had received this stamp of approval in the literature they produced to describe themselves.

The government was not about to set up its own bureaucracy to administer the Medicare program. Instead it agreed to pay an administrative fee to organizations that were already processing health insurance claims. It seemed like a good idea to give that responsibility to an insurance company that was a nonprofit organization rather than one that would make a profit on public funds spent by the government. In time, the for-profit insurance companies convinced the government that they could provide the same services for less. That argument appealed to the government and was popular with the public. Insurance carriers, who bid on providing this service for the lowest fee, now handle Medicare reimbursement claims, generally on a regional basis.

After the first two or three years, the government realized that Medicare costs would not drop as policy analysts had expected. Policy analysts who projected costs had reasoned that a backlog of untreated illness would push up the initial costs of Medicare and Medicaid but that once that backlog was addressed costs would drop. The government did not take major steps to reduce

Medicare costs until 1983, when Diagnostic Related Groups (DRGs) were introduced. The government developed a reimbursement schedule based on the diagnoses with which patients were admitted to the hospital. Hospitals were fully aware that this was coming and knew that the government was using the data that the hospitals themselves were submitting in order to receive Medicare reimbursements to construct the schedule. Amazingly, all possible diagnostic categories were subsumed into 467 categories, plus a few more catchall categories. The system was set up so that the government would pay X amount of money per diagnostic category (one of the 476) per Medicare patient admission. Private insurance companies did not change their reimbursement arrangements in response to the introduction of DRGs, at least not immediately. However, over the decades of the 1990s, private insurance companies adopted the DRG reimbursement schedule and Medicaid programs in most states did, too.

The introduction of DRGs marked an important turning point in the operations of hospitals. Consider the fact that, prior to DRGs, Medicare and all other insurers paid hospitals on the basis of *charges, not costs.* In other words, whatever the hospital charged was what they paid. The government created DRGs, because many critics repeatedly pointed out that paying on a charge, rather than cost, basis was one of the main reasons behind the escalation of costs. They argued that hospitals could and should become more efficient and accountable for how they were spending public funds.

The incentive for hospitals to become more efficient was that if the hospital could do whatever was necessary for less than the DRG payment for particular procedures or services, it got to keep the extra funds. If the funds were insufficient, the hospital simply had to find a way to deal with that. Hospitals did find ways to deal with it. One was to increase charges to patients covered by private insurance. Another way was to begin cutting back on the number of days (*length of stay*) a person stayed in the hospital. In 1980, people were staying in the hospital an average of 7.5 days; by 2007, they were staying 4.8 days.[5]

This strategy did not go unnoticed. The public responded by putting pressure on legislators to pass laws to prevent patients from being discharged earlier than the public thought appropriate, or as policy analysts put it, "quicker and sicker." By the end of 1996, twenty-nine states had passed laws governing "early discharge" to prevent a woman who had just had a baby from being discharged in less than two days or those who had a mastectomy from being discharged the same day.[6] The laws were actually directed at the insurance companies that were imposing restrictions on length of stay.

What do you think: was this a good way to control rising costs? Health policy types saw this as a very strange way to deal with the problem of quality of care. Do we expect state legislators to pass laws to cover every possible concern about hospital care expressed by the public?

Hospitals came up with a number of other ways to make up for the lost earnings they sustained because of tighter Medicare controls. They were already reducing the length of stay—all they had to do was extend that idea. They simply admitted patients for less than a full day (i.e., less than twenty-four hours). Since DRGs cover *inpatient* care but not *outpatient* care, hospitals could charge rates that were not so closely monitored for those patients. That explains why hospitals began building freestanding, outpatient clinics both near and far from the parent hospital.

At about this time a number of other factors came into play that contributed to further reducing the length of stay in the hospital. Surgical techniques had been improving all along, more laser surgery was being used (which is less invasive and may be done on an outpatient basis), and everyone agreed that it was better for the patient to go home to more familiar and comforting surroundings (where there was less chance of contracting new strains of hospital-based infection). Length of stay has a big impact on hospital *occupancy rates*. If people stayed in the hospital for fewer days, that would leave beds empty. If this trend continued hospitals would have to take beds out of service permanently. That is exactly what happened. Some hospitals had such a low "census" or occupancy rate that they could no longer survive.

The upshot of these trends is that hospitals were now admitting more patients who were too seriously ill to be treated on an outpatient basis. This manifested itself in two diametrically opposed trends that actually make perfect sense when you think about it. First, hospitals had no alternative but to increase the ratio of staff to patients; second, personnel costs were steadily declining compared to other hospital costs, which were skyrocketing. What accounts for rising hospital costs is not so difficult to understand once you realize how much new technology hospitals were investing in. This includes diagnostic and monitoring equipment like CT (computerized axial tomography) scanners, MRI (magnetic resonance imaging) equipment, PET (positron emission tomography) scanners, and the computers that compile and analyze all the information that the diagnostic equipment produces. All those machines are enormously expensive, and they are replaced every few years as newer, improved versions are released. Of course, every patient wants the most recent version of any diagnostic instrument available, and your doctor certainly feels that way, too; that, among other things (like the threat of malpractice suits for using outdated equipment) convinces the hospital that staying current is a wise investment.

In order to cover these costs, hospitals increasingly began relying on a very old and familiar funding mechanism, namely, the "sliding scale," meaning the rich pay more. In its more recent incarnation, it became known as "cost-shifting," that is, charging privately insured patients more than those whose bills were paid by public insurance, because public insurance programs reimburse hospitals at a lower rate than private insurance and make every effort to monitor those expenditures. More recently hospitals have been entering into contractual arrangements with some private insurance companies to provide services at reduced rates. Anyone who is not included in such arrangements is charged more. Whether patients who are not covered by such arrangements are actually able to pay what they are charged is another matter.

Unfair? Hospital representatives say that they must take care of persons who carry no insurance but run up high costs. Where are they supposed to get the funds to cover that? Laws passed in 1986 prevent hospitals from turning away patients who are uninsured and unable to pay for care.[7] Therefore, people who had no other regular source of care began coming to emergency rooms with minor as well as major problems, because they knew they would not be turned away even if they could not pay for the care they received.

Hospitals are allowed to stabilize the patients who cannot pay for their care in the emergency room before sending them off, ideally to the nearest "safety-net" hospital. However, this sometimes involves emergency surgery and days spent in the most expensive part of the hospital, the "intensive care" unit. Surgical patients who are admitted to the hospital for a planned, routine surgery typically only spend a short period of time there. Patients who are involved in serious accidents or have multiple gunshot wounds stay much longer.

Some hospitals treat many more poor patients than other hospitals. Recognizing this, the government instituted an adjustment, the "disproportionate share hospital payment," to help community hospitals in poor communities, that is, safety net hospitals, cover their costs a few decades ago. There are a number of ways to meet the disproportionate share hospital (DSH) designation. One criterion is that 30 percent or more of the hospital's patients must be poor enough to qualify for government health insurance. Hospitals that treat 15 percent or more patients who meet this qualification are eligible for a slightly lower DSH subsidy. The majority of hospitals in this country have been receiving DSH payments. The fact that more people lost insurance coverage during the Great Recession meant that hospitals were providing more uncompensated care than ever. The American Recovery and Reinvestment Act of 2009, passed to help the country deal with the problems caused by the recession, increased DSH payments by 2.5 percent.

The recession has had a rather dramatic effect on hospitals. According to the Agency for Healthcare Research and Quality (AHRQ), which operates under the auspices of the U.S. Department of Health and Human Services, hospital stays for uninsured patients increased by 21 percent between 2003 and

2008.[8] By contrast, the total increase in hospital stays was 4 percent. The average cost per uninsured hospital stay was $7,300. Can you see why the hospital sector would be interested in seeing health care reform passed that would reduce the chances that uninsured people would require hospitalization?

GROWTH OF THE FOR-PROFIT HOSPITAL SECTOR

Policy experts became interested in the effects of the steady expansion of for-profit hospitals several decades ago. The representatives of the for-profit hospital corporations argued that what they were doing was socially beneficial because it put pressure on nonprofit hospitals to be more efficient, which, they said, would bring down prices. Critics countered by arguing that the for-profit hospital corporations employed tactics that deserved greater scrutiny. And that closer scrutiny indicates that the for-profit hospitals are not necessarily more efficient. They simply charge more, provide less charitable care, and operate with lower patient-staff ratios. They have lower personnel costs, which they achieve by replacing nurses with advanced training with hiring less expensive, easily replaced "technicians" trained to do very specific tasks (e.g., take blood pressure or give "shots"). When some of the nonprofit hospitals tried this tactic they found that bringing in less skilled personnel increases the risk of mistakes—medication errors, inability to recognize indicators that something is not right, carelessness about disposal of infectious materials, and so on. The only reason the for-profit hospitals could take advantage of this tactic was that they were located in areas where they would attract patients who were less seriously ill, would have a shorter length of stay, which would make them less likely to be at risk of exposure to mistakes.

The larger problem, according to some observers, was that the new more aggressive business practices introduced by the for-profit hospital chains eventually led to mergers and buyouts of smaller for-profit hospital organizations. Hospital corporations were acting more like other businesses. Those who favored the continued growth of the for-profit hospital sector said that it was about time that nonprofit hospitals learned to apply what are recognized to be basic business practices. Critics countered that the for-profits were skimming off the richest, healthiest patients, were doing almost no research, no medical education, and had as their primary goal financial gain benefiting hospital executives and shareholders. The critics went on to argue that the health care delivery system should not be making a profit on the members of society who have the misfortune of being sick. When the FBI charged two of the leading for-profit chains with fraud and very publicly raided their offices during the early years of the twenty-first century—for overcharging Medicare and performing unnecessary surgery—critics said that no one should be surprised because the for-profit approach manifested such behavior.

Cost and Quality of Care

Many agencies under the auspices of the state and federal governments come in to monitor specific activities that go on in the hospital—agencies that oversee food quality, structural standards, billing procedures, and so on. The Joint Commission carries out periodic reviews. A recent study reports that the measures being used by leading agencies may be seriously undercounting adverse events.[9] The researchers said that relying on self-report records is not good enough. They recommend using real-time observation and ongoing electronic record review. The Centers for Medicare and Medicaid took up the challenge.

The Centers for Medicare & Medicaid Services in cooperation with the Hospital Quality Alliance created a consumer-oriented web site called Hospital Compare to track and report hospital errors. It released its first report in March of 2011. The Hospital Quality Alliance is a public-private collaboration that involves a wide range of organizations, including organizations that represent consumers, hospitals, employers, accrediting groups, and doctors in addition to federal agencies. The value of the report depends on the accuracy of the information. Hospitals have identified errors in the reports but generally agree that assessment serves as a useful tool that helps to pinpoint problems.

Preventable error is a serious matter. It has obvious implications for patient health and safety. It also has cost implications. One recent review indicates that the top ten preventable errors account for over two-thirds of the $17.1 billion in costs associated with such errors.[10] Reports on mechanisms designed to identify and track hospital error continue to attract attention.[11]

Then there is the study analyzing a decade of cost and quality outcomes for more than 2.5 million patients at 208 hospitals in California.[12] Researchers report that the hospitals that spent more had lower in-hospital mortality rates for Medicare patients. The average cost of hospital care for patients that did well was $21,072, which is four times more than the cost of care at the lowest-spending hospitals. That does make one consider all the attention being directed at lowering the cost of hospital care and increasing efficiency from a different perspective, doesn't it?

OTHER HEALTH CARE ORGANIZATIONS

Applying one of the basic differentiating characteristics that we used in discussing hospitals, we can differentiate some other health care organizations by whether they care for patients who are *ambulatory* (to ambulate is to walk) or *bedridden*. Ambulatory patients may receive care at clinics, now more often called health centers, which can be freestanding or attached to a hospital. They can be acutely (but temporarily) ill or chronically ill; in both cases they receive health care services on an outpatient basis, for whatever time it takes, meaning a long-term or short-term basis. Persons who may not really be sick but are no longer able to get to the hospital or clinic on a regular basis without a great deal of assistance may end up being admitted to a facility to receive care as inpatients.

Let's focus on health centers or clinics first. Most people who have private insurance see doctors in their offices, which may be located in a building near a hospital and occupied by a long list of doctors. That does not mean that the doctors are part of a health center organization. Health centers or clinics on the other hand are generally located in poor communities and are there to serve patients who are uninsured or have public insurance—in other words as safety-net health care providers.

Health centers receive support from the Health Resources and Services Administration (HRSA), a unit that operates under the auspices of the U.S. Department of Health and Human Services, created in 1980 by the Carter administration. HRSA provides funding through grants for which the health center must apply to become designated as Federally Qualified Health Centers (FQHCs). The centers must show that they are serving a medically underserved population in a particular community that may include migrant workers, homeless residents, or residents of public housing. Centers that meet the criteria for this designation but have not applied for it are known as look-alike centers. They qualify for some of the benefits but not all.

The centers must be governed by a community board representing the population being served. The centers must have a sliding scale fee system in place based on family size and income. The FQHC designation comes with certain benefits. For example, they may purchase drugs at reduced cost, vaccines are provided for uninsured children at no cost and the centers serve as sites where National Health Service Corps (NHSC) medical, dental, and mental health providers may work and receive educational loan repayment (up to $170,000) at no cost to the centers, and providers who work there are provided malpractice insurance by the federal government. FQHCs seem to be doing exactly what they were created to do. Is everyone satisfied to see this happening? We will get back to that.

Turning to long-term care facilities, we find that long-term care has been attracting a considerable amount of attention for some time as the baby boom generation came ever closer to its golden years. As we have already noted, that time has finally arrived with 2011 marking the first year that baby boomers turn sixty-five. And as we have also noted as the boomers develop health problems associated with aging they are expected to break the bank; and, that the list of threatened institutions is lengthy: social security, Medicare, nursing homes, and all associated services required by the elderly.

Added to the increasing number of people who will need nursing home care because of the problems associated with aging, there is the devastation that chronic illness in younger populations causes, for example, developmental disabilities, paralysis due to spinal injury, mental problems, and so forth. Finally, the fact that modern medicine can perform miracles in saving people who would not have survived years ago does not necessarily mean that those who are saved can lead normal, healthy lives. Many require extensive care for years.

Home health care has been supported, in fact promoted, albeit with some trepidation, by the government as a good alternative to nursing home care. The reason that home health care is not likely to be promoted even more enthusiastically is that poses a potential cost problem that is interesting to reflect upon. Home health care is much less expensive than nursing home care because people stay in their own homes and health workers go in for a few hours at a time. Also, virtually everyone prefers to stay in his or her own home. The fear is that too many people will opt for this form of care. Traditionally, wives, daughters, and other female relatives provided such care out of sense of duty. Now that the majority of women are not staying home, the government is concerned that it will have to pick up the bill. For now, the costs do not seem to be rising too rapidly but this cost item is being carefully monitored.

Hospices are another interesting innovation. For years, critics said terminally ill patients did not have to be in the hospital. It was too expensive; it put the patient through unnecessary pain and aggravation; it was a bad idea all around. Hospices promised to provide the patient with comfort and relief from pain, rather than aggressive intervention. The result was expected to be less expensive. As it turns out, the kind of care patients are receiving is pretty much what was anticipated. Most people think it is excellent. The problem is that it has not reduced costs very much.

One of the problems that comes up repeatedly is that the Department of Health and Human Services keeps finding nursing homes in violation of federal health and safety standards. The homes owned by for-profit chains have more violations than either the nonprofit or government-owned nursing homes.[13] The fact that about two-thirds are owned by for-profit companies, 27 percent are nonprofit, and 6 percent are government owned is according to some observers the reason behind the increased risk of violations.

HOSPITALS AND HEALTH CARE REFORM

Hospitals can expect to be seeing an influx of newly insured patients, which will increase revenue as a result of the health care reform law. However, they can also expect some payment reductions. For one, hospitals will be penalized if they have a high rate of potentially preventable readmissions. A list of "never events" has come into existence which identifies mistakes that are so bad that Medicare will not reimburse a hospital for any of the services if a "never event" occurred in the course of treatment. Examples of never events include leaving something inside the patient during surgery or allowing a serious infection to develop at the site of the surgery. Nearly all of the changes are scheduled to take effect by 2014.

An Independent Payment Advisory Board will be convened to recommend policies to reduce Medicare spending if spending exceeds a target growth rate. Disproportionate Share Hospitals will receive reduced payments. Concern about whether nonprofit hospitals really deserve to enjoy freedom from taxes means that the nonprofit hospitals will have to prove that they are providing sufficient community benefit to justify the tax forgiveness. They will have to conduct a community needs assessment every three years and adopt an implementation strategy to address community needs.

One other feature of the ACA may have a far more significant impact. Hospitals will be encouraged to form or participate in Accountable Care Organizations (ACOs). The ACO component was explained in March of 2011, one year after the law was enacted. It is to be launched in 2012. An ACO is envisioned as a network of doctors and hospitals sharing responsibility for patient care. The network would have to agree to manage the care of at least five thousand Medicare beneficiaries for three years or more. Hospitals, doctors, and insurers in some parts of the country began planning to establish ACOs to treat private patients as well as Medicare patients as soon as the law was passed. The rationale behind the law is that the ACOs would be given incentives in the form of bonuses for holding down costs, meeting certain benchmarks for care, and keeping patients out of the hospital.

That sounds pretty good, right? But, the introduction of ACOs is causing a lot of upset. Why? One reason is that hospitals, doctors' groups, and insurers are all competing to set up these networks so they can be in charge. That worries policy makers who are afraid that the participants are rushing in and not spending enough time planning the ventures. Another worry is that if the ACOs really take off, this kind of consolidation might lead to a single health care entity in smaller markets, eliminating any alternative for patients in those areas.

Finally, one very clear rule set forth by the ACA is the prohibition against creation of any new specialty hospitals. Such hospitals have been established by physicians who specialize in performing certain procedures and treating particular kinds of health problems in recent years. The trend started in 2000 when doctors began promoting specialty hospitals they said would employ a "focused factory" approach to treatment. The quality of care was consistently considered to be excellent; patients were highly satisfied. So what's the problem? Critics said that physicians were referring insured, less complicated cases to facilities in which they had a financial interest. This was placing a greater burden on community hospitals to care for the more complicated cases as well as the uninsured patients. The CMS put a moratorium on this development in 2004 but lifted it in 2006 precisely because patients were receiving high-quality care—that plus the fact that doctors were pressing for the right to establish more such hospitals. As it became clear that the ACA would again prohibit specialty hospitals, there was a rush to create new hospitals by the end of 2010. At last count there were two hundred specialty hospitals in existence.

The Questions That Remain

Working backward, are alternatives to hospitalization worth developing further? The general consensus seems to be yes, they are. However, how we can accomplish that is not at all clear. That is where institution building comes in. Since there is no blueprint, anyone who has a plan is trying to institute it. Will that work? No one knows with certainty, but, since we don't know how else to do it, we will most likely continue along the same path. The Accountable Care Organization initiative is such an innovation. We will have to wait to see how that turns out.

How about the future of hospitals? The questions here largely revolve around who we want to see operating them. Asking who is best suited or who will do the best job for us is, at bottom, a matter of perspective on the benefits of competition and private sector ownership as opposed to dependence on nonprofit organizations plus greater government involvement and oversight. This is not something that people debate without emotion. Those who are most closely involved tend to be believers in one approach or the other. Rarely do you find people sitting on the fence. Even if you have not come to this debate with strong feelings about this question already, by the time you finish this book, you too will likely be taking sides. At the heart of the controversy is the question of whether health care organizations are like other organizations that produce and sell goods and services or whether they are somehow different. The argument presented here will come up in almost every chapter.

Medical economists are divided on this question. Some say that health care delivery organizations are special, that they should not be operated for profit. They argue that the misfortune of others should not provide an opportunity to further enrich the rich and powerful in society. And they say that health care is too important to treat as just another commodity that can be traded on the market, like pork bellies, or another product that is purchased as a matter of preference, like a breakfast cereal. Others say that the market offers the best model for the distribution of all goods and services, and that hospitals are no different. Some economists are particularly enthusiastic about the focused factory model of hospitals. It is worth noting that these tend to be economists who are not closely tied to the field of medical economics. They tend to be less interested in analyzing how to deal with complicated cases that require multi-specialty skills and procedures.

Years ago, one economist observed that "a built bed is a filled bed." Given that the rate of hospitalization has declined, hospitals have beds for which they are licensed and which they are reluctant to eliminate. However, it is expensive to maintain unfilled beds and the rooms in which they are located. So hospitals are now doing their best to fill those beds. Should we try to discourage hospitals from pursuing the objective of turning a built bed into a filled bed or will we all benefit if they are innovative about it?

There are obviously many more questions that we could be raising about the direction this sector is going and the impact that the health care reform act will have. Some of those questions will emerge in the chapters on health care personnel, which come next, and the chapters on health insurance, where hospitals get their funding.

· 4 ·

Health Care Occupations

$\mathcal{T}$his chapter focuses on health care occupations, how they developed, and how they have changed over time. The closing section of the chapter outlines how passage of the health care reform act affects health occupations.

The number of people involved in the delivery of health care and the tasks they perform have been steadily increasing. The Bureau of Labor Statistics reports that as of 2011, nearly 11 percent of all the jobs in this country are in the health sector. Consider this figure in contrast to what the health sector looked like a century ago. It is not much of an exaggeration to say that at the beginning of the twentieth century, there were only three positions in the hospital: doctor, nurse, and aide. The doctor's job was to diagnose and treat the patient. Nurses were responsible for keeping the patient clean and comfortable; aides, who may not have been called aides at the time, did the same for everything else in the room. Doctors' offices had no support staff. Sometimes, the doctor's wife would help with the bills, and, of course, someone had to clean the office. How things have changed! Furthermore, this is one of the few parts of the labor force that is predicted to continue expanding, that is, employing even more people in the foreseeable future. This raises a number of basic questions, such as: Where did all those jobs come from? Who is in charge of creating new jobs? How does the work get divided up?

Some 450 occupational titles are involved. Obviously we can only discuss a small number of them. We will devote more attention to doctors, because doctors have the final authority when it comes to diagnosis and treatment, and doctors are licensed to prescribe medications and perform surgery. This is an exclusive right of doctors, with a few notable exceptions such as advanced practice nurses, for example, nurse practitioners, nurse anesthetists, and nurse midwives. Practice privileges vary from state to state. A number of other occupational groups have been challenging doctors' exclusive right to prescribe and treat patients. We will return to this topic at the end of the chapter.

THE MEDICAL PROFESSION

Let's go back to the late nineteenth century to see how medicine as an occupation developed. A number of explanations competed for the existence of ill health, even death, all represented by groups of practitioners who offered a particular set of treatments based on those explanations. There were many kinds of practitioners: hydropaths (who used water to soothe, but more often than not to aggressively heat up or cool down the body); naturopaths (who use natural herbal preparations in prevention and treatment of symptoms); chiropractors (who treat most ailments using back manipulation and massage); homeopaths (who believe in treating "like symptoms with like" in an effort to attain stability and bring comfort); osteopaths or DOs (doctors of osteopathy, who subscribe to the idea that the backbone is the body's control center and that its strength is central to good health); and, allopaths (who engaged in aggressive interventions, such as blood letting and giving emetics to induce vomiting, and if they were not successful, they simply applied more of the same treatment, but were the ones who ultimately succeeded in laying the foundation for mainstream medicine).

By the beginning of the twentieth century, allopathic medicine had firmly allied itself with medical science. The other practitioners did not exactly disappear, although some were absorbed by allopathic, mainstream medicine while others came to be defined as unscientific and lost ground. Practitioners other than mainstream medical doctors now offer what has been called "alternative medicine" or, more recently, "complementary" and "integrative" medicine. The scientific community does not deny that complementary medicine may provide benefits. It is just that the diagnoses and treatments are so individualized that they cannot be standardized or confirmed. What works for one person may not work the same way for another person. Moreover, the medications are not regulated by the Food and Drug Administration. The result is that, as one investigation after another reveals with considerable fanfare, the amount of active ingredient in the medications may or may not be accurate, and may not even be there at all. Yet, some people continue to swear by these products and until a scandal occurs, severe injury or death of a number of people, no one demands that better controls be instituted. And after a while, the whole issue dies down again.

What is it about allopathic medicine that is different, that made it scientific? And why did that allow the allopaths to win the battle of competing explanations for illness and death (i.e., morbidity and mortality respectively)? Being "scientific" simply means that the explanations, and, ultimately, the treatments, allopathic medicine was offering at the end of the nineteenth century could be substantiated. The allopaths could predict the course of disease with and without treatment. The same was true from one instance or one person to another. They verified their diagnoses by doing autopsies. This allowed doctors to compare the symptoms outlined in the patient's file to the effect on the organs involved. They built up a body of knowledge and learned to apply it. An increasing number of people began to believe in their explanations as evidence of their success began to accumulate. Or, if you prefer, the allopaths made every effort to make sure people heard about their successes and were impressed by them.

The larger context of the times in which all this was taking place is worth reflecting on for a moment. This was happening at about the same time that Americans had suddenly become convinced that science was the way to go in all areas of life. During the first decade of the twentieth century there was talk about scientific solutions for such unlikely pursuits as housewifery (i.e., housekeeping) and such popular ones (in some circles) as scientific management. The growth of confidence in scientific medicine was not a unique phenomenon but rather a part of a broader shift in social values and expectations.

Accordingly, when the allopaths (hereafter referred to as doctors or MDs) focused on one area of practice, that is, chose to specialize in treatment of that part of the body, they received high praise and recognition. Patients who could afford it were eager to be treated by medical specialists. True, the vast majority of people could not afford the kind of care medical experts could provide. They relied on home remedies and elixirs provided by the corner druggist. Admittedly, preference for treatment by specialists was something the social elite could indulge in and the middle class made every effort to emulate, and which the poor pretty much ignored because they could not afford to be treated by a doctor, let alone a specialist.

MEDICAL SPECIALIZATION

Let's consider the matter of specialization in more detail. It is worth going back to the late nineteenth and early twentieth century again in order to get the full picture. The first specialty to emerge was ophthalmology (medical and surgical treatment of the eye). One reason for this might be that new and better tools were becoming available during the latter half of the nineteenth century, making it easier to detect abnormalities in the eye. By the late 1800s small groups of doctors were meeting to discuss their observations about the eye and the new tools they were just getting accustomed to using. They were the ones who decided to establish a specialty of their own. Why do that? Was the chance to make more money a primary motivation here? A closer look at how people entered into most occupations might help answer that question.

At the turn of the century one announced his or her occupation by putting up a sign declaring the kinds of work he (mostly he) was prepared to do. City directories, which were much like our current telephone books, listed people's occupations. You could list any occupation you wanted, qualified or not. People could, and did, simply pick up, move, and start doing different kinds of work whenever it suited them. This might be surprising but, until the last decades of the nineteenth century, there was strong opposition to all forms of licensure. When the movement to institute licensure took hold in the 1880s, it occurred on a state-by-state basis. Today states continue to control licensure, and a license from one state may not be honored in another state.

Returning to our ophthalmology example, why would an individual be interested in developing an official specialty designation? After all, anyone who had a medical degree, and, in some cases, those who did not, could put up a sign saying that they specialized in treating diseases of the eye. On the other hand, no one would want to let just anybody treat their eyes. But wasn't insisting that practitioners be required to have a medical license enough? People wanted to be assured that they were going to practitioners who really had the best skills at the time when it came to treating something like the eye. The doctors who were restricting their practices to treating people's eye problems and meeting with colleagues to upgrade their knowledge on a regular basis did in fact know more about eye disease than anyone else. They actually did have greater expertise in their field, but there was no sure way for them to distinguish themselves from anyone else who laid claim to the label of eye specialist.

It was the experts in treatment of eye diseases who decided to institute specialty "certification." The doctors themselves set up training programs and a qualifying test for the purpose of recognizing new practitioners as qualified specialists. Thus, in 1916, ophthalmology became the first certified specialty. As an aside, how do you think other physicians reacted to this event? They were generally pleased, as most reputable doctors were not interested in treating eye problems because the eye is such a complex organ.

Other areas of specialization followed. The majority of doctors continued to identify themselves as general practitioners throughout the first half of the twentieth century. Why is it so difficult to find a general practitioner now and why do we have so many specialists at this time?

World War II stands as a major turning point in how medicine developed in this country, including specialized medicine. The wartime draft made a major impression on doctors. Specialists entered into military service as captains while the general practitioners entered as lieutenants. Obviously, with the higher rank of captain came higher pay and other privileges. Not the least of the privileges was the fact that captains were assigned to hospitals away from the battleground, while the lieutenants were assigned to field hospitals at the front.

A related trend was taking off at home. Because wartime wages were frozen, the only way that companies could make themselves more attractive to prospective employees, who were in short supply, was to offer better benefits. Insurance companies could not operate without standardizing the fees they would pay for the medical services. Prior to this time, doctors pretty much decided what to charge depending on where they practiced and how much their patients were able to pay. It was the insurance companies that set up standardized fee schedules and set the pattern of paying specialists at a higher rate than general practitioners.

Once the war ended, there is the effect of the GI Bill to consider. One of the big rewards for military service during the war was free education upon return. A large number of veterans took advantage of this benefit, including those who already had an MD degree. They went on to get more education and experience better suited to treating patients who were not war casualties. With more training, they became eligible for certification as specialists. Some went on to take specialty certification exams. Many others announced that they were specialists based on the fact that they completed all the requirements and were qualified to take certification tests even if they did not actually take that final step. How did society react? Clearly, people were eager to be treated by doctors who had the most knowledge and expertise, that is, those who were trained as specialists.

Continuing to take a historical perspective, we find that the central feature of life in the United States from the mid-1960s through the early 1970s, in addition to the Vietnam War, anti-war protests, and the civil rights movement, was the increased role that the government was playing in civilian life. The government was funneling considerable sums of money into programs of all kinds—education, housing, social welfare—with medical research receiving a fair share of those funds. Research monies went to medical schools for the purpose of performing specific kinds of research. There was an explosion of scientific knowledge. Medical students were not at all sure that they could learn everything they needed to know. Specialization allowed them to learn more about one subject area. Furthermore, medical students were heavily influenced by the excitement surrounding the work of specialists and super-specialists. Medical faculty served as impressive role models for new trainees.[1]

In the meantime, with all the emphasis on specialization, general practitioners were becoming unhappy. They were being paid less than specialists for providing many of the same services. Patients were referring themselves to specialists because they perceived specialists to be more knowledgeable. The general practitioners decided that they were tired of being treated like second-class citizens. They decided to make themselves specialists in "family practice." In 1971, family practice became a specialty just like any other medical or surgical specialty. After finishing medical school and receiving their MDs, doctors continued their training in specialized residency programs. Prior to this time, a person with an MD was required to complete a one-year internship program in order to obtain a license to practice, granted by the state. From 1971 forward, all MDs would be required to complete residencies lasting at least three years, more to become even more highly specialized. In short, as of 1971, MDs could no longer become general practitioners. Over the next few decades, smaller numbers of MDs were opting to train as family practitioners. Doctors receiving the Doctor of Osteopathy degree, DOs, now serve as the country's family practitioners. DOs can go on for specialty training by entering into residency programs offered by MD medical schools.

We now refer to doctors who are primarily responsible for a patient's health as "primary care" practitioners or as the latest acronym would have it, as PCPs. This includes internists, pediatricians, and family practitioners.

MEDICAL ERROR AND MALPRACTICE

Coincidently, just about the time that the general practice option was abolished, Americans began to register increasing dissatisfaction with their health care arrangements. They complained that doctors were no longer interested in the whole person; that they were only interested in treating parts of the person; and that they were only doing it for the money. Why this did not happen previously when doctors could do so much less for their patients is not hard to understand when you consider that over previous decades, the majority of doctors were general practitioners who were located in the community where their patients lived. Members of the community got to know the doctor. When they needed to see the doctor, they went with the added comfort of an established sense of familiarity and trust. That is not the case when patients see a specialist for a specific problem on a one-time basis. When things go wrong, it is a lot easier to sue that doctor, who is, after all, a stranger. This explains, in part, the high rate at which patients are suing doctors for malpractice these days.

A number of other factors, including the rising size of settlements, may have contributed to what has come to be viewed as a malpractice crisis during the early years of the twenty-first century. Some observers believe that the widely quoted report on the rate of medical error has something to do with it. The matter of medical error came to public attention in 1999 when the Institute of Medicine (IOM, the quasi-government organization created to advise the nation on health issues) reported that 44,000 to 98,000 people die in hospitals per year due to preventable error.[2] While the numbers were actively disputed, everyone agreed that error reduction was a highly laudable objective. The IOM report also clearly stated that the rate of error was due to systemic failure rather than malpractice on the part of doctors. Nevertheless, it is possible that the report prompted some dissatisfied patients to sue.

There is no reliable count of the number of malpractice suits that are filed per year, their outcome, or the awards. Researchers who have studied this issue focus largely on the impact malpractice has had on health care spending.[3] The best estimate available at present is that the country spent about $55.6 billion, or 2.4 percent of total health care expenditures, in 2008 on awards, legal expenses, the extra expense of defensive medicine, and other costs that are hard to calculate such as lost time, reputational harm, and subsequent price increases.

The topic began receiving attention from policy analysts a decade or so ago because jury awards were becoming enormous and were rising faster than economic growth could explain. The median jury award in 1997 was $500,000, jumping to $1,010,858 in 2002, even though the proportion of cases won by plaintiffs, 42 percent, remained the same.[4] Doctors were most concerned about the major effect the payout level was having on the malpractice insurance premiums they would have to pay. By 2002, the average annual premium in the southern part of Florida (the highest in the country) for obstetricians/gynecologists was $211,000; for surgeons it was $124,000; and for internists it was $56,000.[5] Obstetricians are at a particularly high risk of being sued. Those who monitor these things say that they are sometimes sued not because they did something wrong, but because parents want to blame someone if their baby is not perfect. The solution that emerged over time is "tort reform."

Tort reform has a very specific meaning in this context; it refers to instituting a ceiling on the award for "pain and suffering." This ceiling or cap does not affect recovery of the cost of the medical treatment related to the event, the cost of care in the future, and future lost income. California was the first state to impose the cap at $250,000. The fact that the lowest malpractice premiums for internists can be found in California at $3,200 and highest in states that do not have a cap, for example $48,245 in Florida and $41,066 in Illinois in 2011 has convinced doctors that the cap provides an important solution to their problem.[6]

Malpractice lawyers argue that suing doctors is the best approach for protecting patients from incompetent doctors because the threat of being penalized makes doctors more careful. Doctors argue that lawyers are motivated to sue even when there is no evidence of error because they stand to collect one-third of the settlement if they go to court and win and one-fourth if the case is settled out of court. They take cases on "contingency," that is, they get paid if they win and get paid nothing if they lose. Lawyers argue that this allows people who could not possibly afford to hire a lawyer and pay all the costs involved in a trial to be represented.

For their part, insurance companies are willing to settle out of court on a batch of suits even when there is no evidence of medical error in order to avoid the cost of going to court. The settlements, in turn, raise malpractice premium costs for all doctors in the insurance pool and leave an undeserved blemish on doctors' records whose cases were settled without any effort to check to see whether the claims had any validity to them. Some doctors have countersued and won. However, that takes more time, effort, and money than most are willing to expend.

Policy analysts have yet another take on the issue. They say that it is not an issue to which they are willing to devote much attention. They point out that because malpractice insurance premiums amount to only 2 percent of national spending, tort reform would have little effect on the total health care bill.[7] Physicians disagree. They argue that they are forced to practice defensive medicine, that is, order tests they know are not really necessary in order to avoid the accusation that they did not do everything possible to treat the patient. That clearly increases costs. Policy analysts agree that this is a widespread pattern, but they maintain that defensive medicine has less impact on costs than doctors would like to believe.

So what do policy analysts say is the most promising solution for reducing the risk of malpractice? Many argue that the solution is continued medical education for doctors and safety checklists for hospitals. Safety checklists have had a major effect on reduction of hospital-based error and infection. Counting instruments in the surgical suite before closing up the patient eliminates one clearly avoidable error. Hand washing and using hand sanitizer has had an enormous impact on reducing hospital-based infections, which are especially difficult to treat once patients are exposed to them. It is not difficult to see why policy analysts would argue that taking such steps produces significant social benefit even if it does not reduce costs.

One more initiative is designed to reduce risk of mistakes related to paperwork if not medical practice. The Obama administration set aside $19 billion dollars in the economic recovery act of 2009 to provide incentives for doctors to install electronic medical records software. The incentive comes in the form of a $40,000 payment to physicians who initiate electronic record keeping. While most people agree this will help prevent prescription and treatment errors, it has been an uphill battle. The problems start with finding the right software, then getting everyone in the office trained to use it, then coordinating it with all the other offices, including hospital departments, then deciding who will contribute data, and, finally, linking all this to billing. Eventually tracking patient treatment outcomes will be made much more efficient, but this is not happening with lightning speed. We will return to the topic of malpractice reform in the concluding chapter to explore further the implications of malpractice reform.

THE MEDICAL EDUCATION SYSTEM

Let's consider the historical development of medical schools in this country. Considering that, prior to the twentieth century, anyone who was interested in setting up a medical practice could do so without the need to prove competence permitted a wide range of medical training arrangements, including apprenticeships with no coursework, no books, and no labs. Clearly, this was not the best way to learn about the practice of medicine. The "medical establishment" (that is code for organized medicine or the American Medical Association [AMA] and its affiliates, the state and local medical societies) had been aware of this situation ever since the middle of the nineteenth century. However, the people who ran these inferior schools were colleagues and fellow AMA members. The issue was a delicate one. Most doctors weren't making a great deal of money treating patients especially in communities that were not wealthy (remember there were no insurance companies that would guarantee payment in those days). Training fees were an important source of income. Telling colleagues that they would no longer be allowed to accept such fees because the schools they were operating were inferior was not a topic that other doctors wanted to broach.[8]

The situation was resolved without much input from the majority of people in society. The elite members of the AMA shared their concerns with others in their social circle, confident that such information would not be passed on to the wrong people (i.e., the public). This is when the Carnegie Foundation became interested in the problem. The Carnegie Foundation was (and still is) devoted to improving education at all levels. In 1907, it took on the task of improving the quality of medical education. The person who was invited to assume responsibility for this assignment was Abraham Flexner.

Flexner visited all 186 medical schools and training programs in existence at the time with the aim of rating them. He was welcomed because the Carnegie Foundation was known to distribute funds to schools. It was not until 1910, just before the Flexner Report was due to be released, that it became clear what Flexner was doing.[9] He graded all the schools he visited on a scale of A through F. The schools to which he had given an "F" closed down even before the report was out. Others began upgrading immediately. Many could not survive. By 1920, only eighty medical were schools left.

The standard against which Flexner rated all other schools was the Johns Hopkins Medical School. He used Johns Hopkins as a model because it grounded its coursework in a scientific body of knowledge rather than in practical experience gained through apprenticeship. That meant two years of basic science courses before the school allowed students to see a patient under the supervision of a senior doctor. That is obviously an expensive proposition compared to apprenticeship training. It is easy to see why Johns Hopkins was not the first choice for those with limited resources.

The Flexner Report had a number of effects. It eliminated the worst medical schools, which were also the schools that prospective medical students from poor families could afford. That had an effect on the composition of the occupation. It had an effect on the chances of minority students being able to get a medical education. It affected women's medical schools, which lacked resources needed to upgrade. Few women were seeking a medical education in those days, and those who did generally did not come from wealthy families. Medicine also became more science-based. The smaller number of schools meant that fewer students could be accepted, which, in turn, meant that the schools could be more selective. The schools could accept only the most highly qualified applicants, who were, of course, white, male, and from a higher social class.

The quality of medical education is no longer a matter of major concern. There is always some debate about whether the curriculum should include more social science to improve doctors' sensitivity to a range of issues such as cultural differences, comfort discussing risky behaviors, and death and dying, to name a few of those issues. A problem that those most closely connected to the medical profession have been very concerned about over recent decades is the cost of medical education. According to the American Association of Medical Colleges, physicians had an average educational debt in 2009 of $156,456. This is worth keeping in mind when we consider how much money doctors make.

MEDICAL EDUCATION AND THE MEDICAL MODEL

The medical education system, built on a foundation that valued science over other scholarly pursuits, translated into what social scientists saw as the "medical model" perspective on illness. The model explains why doctors are not responsive to patients' complaints that do not fit into a recognizable disease pattern. If the patient's complaint cannot be verified through observable indicators and symptoms, then the problem not only cannot be identified, but, more to the point, it cannot be treated using scientifically grounded practice patterns. Physicians consider this to be obvious. They do not deny that the patients who say that they do not feel well do in fact feel poorly. However, their response is that it is not the province of scientific medical practice. Critics of the "medical model" point out that there are other important dimensions to being sick. After all, a person might have a fatal disease and not know it and not seek treatment and not even act sick. Other people may know how sick they are, but choose to work and fulfill other responsibilities as if they were in excellent health. And then there are people who feel tired, headachy, and nauseous who test out as perfectly healthy. Who is and who is not sick in such cases? Doctors say they need objective proof of the presence of illness and disease in the form of indicators signaling some abnormality.

Whether we agree with their assessment or not, doctors decide who is and who is not sick. This matters more than it might at first appear. Sick-day policies at the workplace depend on it. Whether students are allowed to take makeup exams often depends on such information. In general, a doctor's diagnosis pretty much determines whether one gets sympathy for being sick or whether one is treated as if one is whining unnecessarily. Having no good alternative, we end up relying on doctors to say whether someone is sick or not. If a person can present a label assigned by a doctor, then that person is much more likely to be treated as if he or she is really sick and deserves to be excused for not meeting normal deadlines and responsibilities. In short, doctors have a great deal of power to define things by assigning socially acceptable labels. This raises the question of whether this power is more beneficial or more harmful to us as patients and to society as a whole. Logic requires that critics offer an alternative. That's where things fall apart. There does not seem to be much consensus regarding possible alternatives to the medical model other than saying that there are other dimensions to being sick than the ones that doctors can objectively identify, and that an individual's sense of those dimensions should count for more than it does.

DOCTORS AND THE ISSUE OF MONEY

Given all the complaints about doctors, why is it that we as a society continue to pay them so much money? Let's look at how much they earn. In order to get a more detailed picture, let's look at the earnings of a selected category

Table 4.1.   Physicians' Earnings in 2010

Pediatric endocrinology	$187,957
Family medicine	208,861
Internal medicine	214,307
Gynecology & Obstetrics	275,152
General surgery	357,091
Anesthesiology	370,500
Orthopedic surgery	500,672
Cardiac & Thoracic surgery	533,084
Orthopedic surgery—Joint replacement	605,953
Orthopedic surgery—Spine	688,503

Data from "Physician Compensation Survey," The American Medical Group Association, Alexandria, VA (online at www.cejkasearch.com/view-compensation-data/physician-compensation-data/#).

of specialists. Table 4.1 shows income based on a compensation survey by a leading health occupations search firm. These are median incomes (i.e., the halfway point between the lowest and the highest levels of income). That means that some doctors earn a great deal less and some earn a great deal more.

Remember that doctors' net income is considerably lower than their practice revenue because they must pay malpractice premiums and pay off educational loans. Would you agree that that there is so much variation in earnings, it makes it harder to lump all doctors together into one income category? Beyond that, can you see a pattern? Without question, surgeons who perform highly specialized kinds of surgery are now and have traditionally been the high earners.

There's more to the matter of how much doctors are reimbursed for their services. The fees that doctors receive are largely set by the government, specifically by the Centers for Medicare & Medicaid Services (CMS), an agency that operates under the auspices of the U.S. Department of Health and Human Services. Even though Medicare is a program that is basically for persons who are over sixty-five, the government spends so much on Medicare that it has reason to be interested in establishing controls over the monies it pays out to doctors. Remember, that is why Medicare established the DRGs that govern hospital reimbursement. In 1992 it established something called the Resource Based Relative Value Scale (RBRVS) fee schedule for reimbursing doctors. Actually a team of economists from Harvard University worked it out in consultation with doctors and a variety of interested parties over a period of about four years. There were no surprises when it went into effect. The RBRVS schedule calculated a fee for every procedure that doctors perform. The CMS announces how much it will increase and/or decrease fees every year. The battle is waged in Congress. Each year CMS announces what Congress has set as the adjustment or reduction. Shortly after that, Congress passes a bill that adjusts the fee schedule so that the fees do not decline. The health care reform bill addresses the topic of physician reimbursement, which we will examine later in this chapter.

Until the last few decades, the majority of doctors in this country were in private practice or fee-for-service practice. According to the Bureau of Labor Statistics only 12 percent of physicians were self-employed as of 2009; 19 percent were employed by hospitals; and the remaining 53 percent were under contract working in physicians' offices.

Before we go further, let's return for a moment to the fact that such a small proportion of physicians are self-employed. Doctors worked very hard to gain society's respect by embracing a set of practices that they presented as "medical professionalism." In fact, medicine became the model "profession" that many other occupations made every effort to emulate in order to gain some of the privileges that professionalism was providing to doctors including respect, trust, high income, and access to the person's body and to personal information related to illness. The most central feature of medical professionalism was the understanding that the physician would be directly responsible to the patient, rather than to some third party that could stand between the patient and the doctor. This was firmly embedded in the fee-for-service arrangement. The AMA and its state affiliates were adamant about this. The AMA did not object to medical faculty taking salaried positions because they were primarily engaged in research rather than patient care. So now that an increasing proportion of physicians are accepting salaries—what does that say about medical professionalism?

Indeed, does this mean that they will soon be joining unions to negotiate as a group rather than as individuals?[10] And where does that leave all those other occupations that were so committed to emulating the model of professionalism set forth by physicians? It is worth noting that physicians in private practice, who stood as model professionals for so long, are actually considered small business–persons for legal purposes and are therefore prohibited by law from bargaining collectively, that is, joining unions. Will the shift in employment status change the way they see themselves and their ability to negotiate over wages and benefits with increasingly larger and more powerful health care organizations? It turns out that the topic of professionalism is relevant to the development of nursing as an occupation to which we turn next.

NURSES

Nursing is the single biggest occupational category in the health sector. According to the Bureau of Labor Statistics there were about 2.6 million nurses in the country in 2009, 60 percent of whom were working in hospitals. Nursing provides an interesting contrast to medicine because it is overwhelmingly a female occupation and because its origins are so different than those of medicine. The history of nursing is heavily influenced by the traditions introduced by Florence Nightingale. Prior to her work during the Crimean War in the 1880s, nursing was not considered a respectable activity for women from good families. It was considered dirty work. Nightingale emphasized the use of skills available to every middle-class young woman, namely, cleaning wounds, changing bandages, and comforting patients. She gained acceptance for nursing as a suitable occupation for a young woman from a respectable family by assuring doctors that nurses were there to assist them, and not get in their way. Therein lay the problem that nursing has faced ever since.

Historically, nursing care was performed by female members of the household largely to care for members of the family who needed such assistance. Only after nursing became an identifiable occupation during the twentieth century did nurses start to work outside the home. Those who worked in the patient's home were called private duty nurses. Their duties were not strictly defined; in addition to nursing care, they ended up doing a little food preparation, a little house cleaning, maybe a little clerical work—whatever the client wanted and the nurse was willing to do.

As hospitals became a more regular source of care during the twentieth century, nurses began doing more work in hospitals. Private duty nursing eventually became defined as less professional. After all, you really didn't have to be a nurse to manage the personal care needs of people who were not acutely ill. As hospitals began caring for more seriously ill patients, nurses needed to have more training.

Nurses' training continued to reflect the philosophy introduced by Florence Nightingale. Nursing schools were opened by hospitals providing something closer to on-the-job training than education with a theoretical base. Nursing students were expected to live in a dorm with strict rules, to be chaperoned, and to perform nursing tasks in the hospital under supervision for three years. Upon graduation they received a diploma and were qualified to take a state-licensing exam leading to working as a Registered Nurse, or RN. The relationship between doctors and nurses is best captured by the fact that nurses were expected to stand up when a doctor walked into the room and not sit until the doctor permitted it.

At some point colleges began instituting bachelor's degrees in nursing. After completing four years of college and successfully passing the state licensure exam, a nursing student became an RN, just like the diploma graduate. During the 1960s, when there was so much interest in advancing health care and increasing the pool of health care personnel, two-year associate-degree nursing programs were created. The graduates of those programs also became RNs. This created a problem. There were now three different routes into nursing, based on different levels of education and experience. In other words, nursing, as an occupation, did not establish control over the educational system and entry into the occupation. More troubling was the fact that the content of nursing programs varied across the three entry routes, but the nurses were largely being treated the same way by hospitals, which became their primary employers, no matter which program they completed.

Anytime hospitals faced a shortage of nurses in the past, hospitals did not address the problem by raising nursing salaries, as would happen in most other occupational sectors; they just recruited more student nurses into their diploma programs. Several decades ago, most hospitals closed down their diploma programs as they realized that on-the-job training was not enough to prepare nurses to care for the more seriously ill patients now being admitted to hospitals. This has not benefited nursing as much as one might expect, because hospitals simply began training other kinds of workers to do specific tasks and aggressively recruiting nurses from other countries.

The fact that nursing has traditionally been a female occupation, that nurses have historically been employees rather than independent practitioners like doctors, and that their training does not take nearly as long as medical school are factors that explain nursing's occupational fate.

The attention that the effect of nursing care on the health outcomes of hospitalized patients has been receiving over the last few years may alter that perspective. There is a body of evidence developing to indicate that more favorable nurse-to-patient ratios, education, and experience all contribute to better patient outcomes.[11] This together with the unremitting shortage of nurses has brought pressure to bear on legislators. California was the first state to pass a statute requiring hospitals to maintain an eight-to-one patient-to-nursing staff ratio in 2003. The conventional wisdom says that what happens in California predicts what will be happening in other parts of the country in the future. That seems to be true in this case. The battle was successfully waged by the California Nurses Association (CNA), which split off from the American Nurses Association (ANA) because the California nurses wanted to negotiate over wages and working conditions. By 2009, the CNA had joined with the National Nurses United, the United American Nurses, and the Massachusetts Nurses Association to form the largest nurses' union in the country. The ANA continued to say unionism is a threat to the perception of nurses as professionals. However, the success of the CNA is hard to dismiss and the ANA has been giving the issue more thought.

One of the steps nursing as an occupation has taken to deal with the problem of professionalism over the last few decades is to carve out niches in which nurses could work more independently. Nursing created a number of "advanced practice" nursing programs, including nurse midwifery (delivering babies), nurse anesthetist programs, and nurse practitioner programs. All of these require master's-degree-level training. In addition, there are doctoral-level programs leading to a Ph.D. or doctorate in nursing practice. Nevertheless, doctors are legally authorized to diagnose, prescribe, and treat patients, while nurses are generally not allowed to do so. Some states give broader practice privileges to nurses, meaning that they permit nurse practitioners to have their own offices and their own patients, but even in those instances, doctors have final authority if questions arise.

Like nurse practitioners, certified nurse midwives are considered to be primary health care providers in certain underserved areas. In urban and suburban communities, nurse midwives work with doctors to manage normal pregnancies. Studies regularly show that women are very satisfied with the care they receive from nurse midwives, probably because nurse midwives allow the women more control over the delivery process, allowing them to take more time to deliver. There is no difference in birth outcomes between deliveries managed by nurse midwives and doctors, which may be due to the fact that nurse midwives are willing to refer high-risk pregnancies to doctors. The question this kind of evidence raises is whether greater reliance on such "physician extenders" should be advocated more vigorously.

Nurses with advanced degrees who work in hospitals typically have managerial responsibilities in addition to patient care responsibilities. They oversee the work of licensed practical nurses (LPNs, who receive anywhere from six months to over a year of training), nurses aides (who receive a few months of training), and unit clerks (who are hired without special training to carry out the secretarial tasks for nurses in a hospital).

Before we move on to another health occupation, do you think the fact that doctors are accepting salaried positions, and continue to be seen as professionals, is influencing what is happening in nursing? Nurses would undoubtedly say that what doctors do is of no concern. However, a bigger social development may be in the making here.

THERAPISTS

A wide range of occupational groups falls under this designation. Two of the most commonly recognized are physical therapists and occupational therapists. Activities therapists (in music or art) work with patients who are hospitalized for longer stays. Then there are also less well-known categories of therapists in hospitals, such as respiratory therapists. Not all therapists work in hospitals; for example audiologists and speech therapists may have private offices and private practices. Additionally, a number of other occupational groups doing psychological counseling call themselves therapists or counselors. In short, therapists come to this work from wide-ranging backgrounds and with a variety of degrees.

TECHNICIANS

Technicians may constitute an even broader category. Medical technicians work in hospital or clinic laboratories. It is hard to tell technicians from technologists, who usually have more education and training than technicians but work in the same lab doing related tasks. X-ray technicians work directly with patients and have been around for a long time. There are now technicians associated with all kinds of new diagnostic equipment whose work is similar to that of X-ray technicians, for example, sonography technicians, mammography technicians, CT technicians, nuclear medicine technicians, and so on. Many new occupational categories came on board in hospitals as hospitals created new jobs and trained people to do particular tasks. For instance, hospitals trained pharmacy technicians to count pills and bottle them, blood technicians to draw patients' blood, and so on. Hospitals can and do take particular tasks and turn them into specific occupations, such as taking a patient's temperature, taking blood pressure, giving patients injections, and so on.

Then there are emergency medicine technicians (EMTs). They attend to people in an ambulance in an emergency situation. Their objective is to stabilize the patient and get him or her to the emergency room. In some ways their work is comparable to that of physicians' assistants in the sense that they take direct responsibility for the patient under the guidance of doctors. In the case of EMTs, they are able to connect patients to equipment that is monitored by doctors in the emergency room. But it is the EMTs who administer treatment.

Physicians' assistants (PAs), who don't actually fit neatly into any one of the designations, perform tasks that a physician assigns to them. Physicians have been employing increasing numbers of PAs in recent years. According to the American Association of Physician Assistants, as of 2008 there were 142 accredited educational programs and 68,124 persons active in the field; over half work in physicians' offices. PAs may also assist in surgery, do continuing care for surgical patients, go on home visits in some parts of the country more than others, and so on. They differ from nurse practitioners in that PAs work under the physician's license, while nurse practitioners work under their own licenses. In other words, the PA may do brain surgery, if the physician who employs him (more often him than her) is willing to accept responsibility (which is not to say that hospitals would be willing to let this happen). There is a movement to change the name from "physician assistant" to "physician associate," which some physicians agree does more accurately reflect the work of these people.

OTHER PRACTITIONERS

There are two categories of practitioners known as "limited practice" doctors. This includes podiatrists, who are licensed to treat the full range of foot ailments, and dentists, who treat teeth and gums. Dentists and podiatrists are licensed to perform surgery and administer medications. They are doctors. These privileges differentiate them from other practitioners, who may also call themselves doctors. An example is optometrists, who are licensed to examine the eye and prescribe lenses, but must refer patients to an ophthalmologist, who is an MD specializing in the treatment of eye disease, when they detect eye disease.

Similarly, pharmacists are licensed to dispense medications but not prescribe them, even though in many instances they know a great deal more about drug interactions than doctors do. In some hospitals, clinical pharmacists with advanced degrees go on "rounds" together with medical staff to explain drug interactions to medical residents.

ADMINISTRATORS AND OTHER ADMINISTRATIVE WORKERS

Hospital administrators generally come to this work with master's degrees in hospital administration or a comparable degree. The degrees are granted by business schools, schools of public health, medical schools, and a variety of other kinds of programs. The coursework is, however, not all that different. Hospital administrators must be prepared to oversee a wide variety of activities and occupational groups in hospitals and all the other kinds of health care delivery settings (e.g., extended care facilities, outpatient facilities, managed care settings, psychiatric hospitals, and so on).

The scope of their responsibility is interesting to consider. Their authority comes from the board of directors or board of trustees, depending on whether the institution is for-profit or nonprofit. They have full authority and responsibility for running the organization on a day-to-day basis. Decisions involving major changes or expenses are the province of the board, and the administrator is responsible for carrying them out. However, one gray area continues to be somewhat less than clear, although more so in the past than at present: the relationship between hospital administrators and doctors.

One of the biggest responsibilities that falls to administrators is overseeing record keeping. And there are records of all kinds—the usual ones such as payroll records and purchasing records, of course; more complicated matters revolve around patients' medical files, insurance records, billing records, and anything that might be required in malpractice cases. Protecting the organization from malpractice is a career in and of itself. In fact, a new occupational role called "risk management" is dedicated solely to eliminating as many opportunities for malpractice suits as possible—from making sure the railings are sturdy enough to hold up patients who need them, to making sure that patients who want to discuss a problem are put in contact with the person with authority over that area.

Hospital medical records departments, where medical records technicians work, has been one of the fastest-growing areas in the health sector because of the vast amount of information to record. And it has changed dramatically. Until the last couple of decades of the twentieth century, medical record keeping was a matter of filing pieces of paper. Now it is a matter of keeping computerized records and worrying about a whole set of new concerns, especially identifying the right filing code, which determines how much third-party payers will pay the hospital. Representatives of government programs have stepped up efforts to identify and reduce overpayment. If they find that the hospital has been underpaid, it is the hospital's loss. This matter clearly will be attracting a lot more attention in the near future.

HEALTH OCCUPATIONS AND HEALTH CARE REFORM

The Affordable Care Act is mandating a number of changes that do not sound extensive when we consider each one separately but when we consider all of them we can see that the cumulative effect is significant.

- A Patient-Centered Outcomes Research Institute is being established to conduct research focusing on clinical effectiveness.
- Five-year demonstration grants are being awarded to states to develop alternatives to tort litigation, i.e., malpractice reform.
- Medicaid payments for primary care services are being increased to 100 percent of the Medicare reimbursement rate.
- Physicians are being invited to create innovation centers to assist in restructuring government program payments while maintaining or improving quality of care.
- An Independent Payment Advisory Board is being established to reduce per capita growth in Medicare spending.

- Funds for the training and development of the health care workforce are being increased.

The Accountable Care Organizations (ACOs) Rule, which we discussed in the last chapter, seems to be a bigger deal for physicians than for hospitals for a number of reasons. To start with, the money involved is impressive. The CMS estimates that start-up costs and first-year expenses will amount to $1.76 million per ACO. Payouts to the 75 to 150 ACOs that are expected to develop could reach $800 million in bonuses over the first three years. CMS also projects collecting $40 million in penalties. Doctors were informed that they could set up ACOs without linking up with a hospital, but of course they would then be shouldering all of the risk. One of the risks has been identified in a joint statement issued by the Department of Justice, the Federal Trade Commission, and the Department of Health and Human Services. The announcement stated that an ACO that grows large enough to provide 50 percent or more of the services in a particular area will come under the scrutiny of these agencies; only those that have 30 percent or less of the market will avoid such scrutiny.[12]

In short, physicians, with or without the cooperation of hospitals, are being encouraged to establish these operations but to avoid becoming too successful at it.

One initiative the law emphasizes is support for connecting patients to a "medical home." The law has appropriated funds available as of 2010 to support the development of "primary care model" medical homes that integrate physical and mental health services and team management of chronic illness. Interestingly, poor people, who are more likely to receive care at health centers and clinics created to care for poor people are, in fact, receiving care in settings that come much closer to being medical homes than people who seek health care from doctors they choose to see. In other words, because middle-class patients decide which doctors they want to see, they are less likely to receive care in a medical home setting than poor people. Given that there is mounting evidence that care provided in a medical home type setting is generally superior to care that most Americans get by seeking care from assorted specialists who do not coordinate care, it is interesting to find that the medical profession has been so slow to adopt the idea and the public has expressed so little enthusiasm about it.

That may have something to do with the negative experience some people had with HMOs. We will be discussing HMOs in greater detail in the following chapter. For now, let's just say that patients who signed up with HMOs were not pleased to find themselves being forced to abandon doctors they had been seeing for a long time and required to see doctors affiliated with the HMO. More upsetting, HMOs were starting up and being sold to larger health corporations so quickly that patients ended up seeing new doctors every time they went. The transition period produced a great deal of dissatisfaction and the traditional fee-for-service arrangement has virtually disappeared. And the cost of health care just kept rising. Some people are concerned that the Accountable Care Organization plan will repeat this pattern, causing more disruption than beneficial change.

A number of initiatives enacted before the ACA was passed are worth noting because they have had an effect on the work of a number of health occupations. For example, legislation enacted under the Bush administration to expand health information technology (IT) was reinforced by the Obama administration through the American Recovery and Reimbursement Act of 2009. The 2009 legislation mandated $19.2 billion to cover enhanced Medicare and Medicaid payments to providers who adopt electronic record keeping. This is proving difficult to put into effect for various reasons—concerns about privacy protection, lack of commonly agreed-upon software, the time and cost of training personnel, and so on.

A number of other problems have been bubbling up which the medical establishment has had to deal with. For example, there is the matter of "freebies." While there are no legislative measures to address the problem, professional organizations such as the AMA, Association of Medical Colleges, and the American College of Physicians have all taken a strong stand on doctors' readiness to accept freebies from pharmaceutical companies. Once the extent of the practice was exposed, there was considerable pressure from the respected spokespersons within medical profession condemning the practice. There is reason to believe that fewer doctors have been accepting gifts from pharmaceutical companies over the last few years.

Another issue the medical establishment confronts on a fairly regular basis is the effort of a range of occupational groups to challenge the exclusivity of its practice privileges. When nurse midwives proceeded to establish birthing clinics in some poor rural areas a couple of decades ago, the medical establishment did not protest too vigorously. What highly trained physician wants to live in a poor rural area?

But when psychologists began lobbying their states to permit them to prescribe drugs, including the most advanced psychotropic drugs, over the last few years, the medical establishment was not so complacent. There are such efforts going on in seven states at the present time.[13] How much education and training does a psychologist need to prescribe psychotropic drugs—is a master's degree enough? Whether the psychologist must collaborate with a physician is another point of debate. Advanced practice nurses in some states are also lobbying to gain the right to establish private practices with all the privileges that doctors now have. Naturopaths in over fifteen states have been arguing with varying success for the right to prescribe medication and deliver babies for the last decade or so.

What do you think? Would having more practitioners providing health care services be a good thing for society and serve a greater number of people who are not currently getting the care they need, or would it produce more problems than it solves?

· 5 ·

Private Health Insurance

$\mathcal{T}$his is where we finally get to the topic of health insurance coverage, which is at the core of the Affordable Care Act. We will begin the chapter with an overview of the origins of health insurance in this country and go on to examine how health insurance has worked over the last eighty years or so. Finally, in the latter half of the chapter we will focus on the alterations the ACA has introduced. There is no question that the measures the law introduces are complicated. However, think of it this way: you will have a better understanding of the law than most Americans and you will be in a position to gloat about that whenever the topic comes up.

Let's begin our assessment of health insurance arrangements by distinguishing between public and private insurance programs. *Public* is code for government-sponsored and supported. *Private* is everything that is not run by the government. Private health insurance comes in two forms: 1) *private, nonprofit* and 2) *private, for-profit*. The difference between nonprofit and for-profit has to do with what happens to the money the organization earns at the end of the year. In for-profit corporations, stockholders, who have invested in the company with the expectation of making money, receive a share of the profits in the form of increased value of the stock they own and, in some cases, payouts called dividends. Nonprofit organizations have no investors and do not earn a "profit." If they take in more than they pay out, the organization puts the "excess" back into the organizational coffers. No one gets to keep any part of the excess as a bonus. The money is used to upgrade the organization's offerings, equipment, programs, and so forth.

While groups of people here and there may have established funds to help each other in times of need, the need to protect against the costs of health care was the a major concern prior to the 1930s. Two very different models of health insurance coverage have come into existence since then. The Great Depression certainly played a role in helping to launch both types of coverage—the Blue Cross–Blue Shield fee-for-service insurance model and the Kaiser Permanente prepaid plan model.

THE FEE-FOR-SERVICE MODEL

The first major insurance plan developed in this country was the Blue Cross plan, which was developed at Baylor University Hospital in Dallas in 1929.[1] The hospital was struggling, like all hospitals during that era, because so many patients could not pay their bills once the Great Depression hit. A review of the records revealed that schoolteachers constituted one clearly identifiable category of people defaulting on their bills. Baylor University Hospital came up with the following plan. It offered the Dallas Board of Education a plan whereby teachers would pay 50 cents a month for twenty-one days of hospital coverage per year. The plan caught on. In fact, it spread across the country. Over the following decade other cities, in many cases whole states, established their own Blue Cross plans, which eventually spawned a Blue Shield addition and became established as Blue Cross–Blue Shield (BC–BS) plans.

The Blue Shield side of the plan evolved more slowly and was not nearly as successful as the Blue Cross side. Blue Shield was created to cover physicians' charges. However, it was more difficult to administer because there were so many doctors and so many different services that it was impossible to standardize rates. (Computers have, of course, solved that problem.) Also, there was no one to champion this cause. Doctors were not nearly as enthusiastic about instituting insurance arrangements for their services as were hospitals.

The features of the Blue Cross side of the plan were considered groundbreaking at the time. First, it was conceived of as a nonprofit plan, meaning that it was designed to cover its costs and not make a profit. Second, in order to ensure that costs, which were largely unpredictable, would be covered, the people instituting the plan came up with an idea that was considered very innovative. The plan called for everyone to pay the same amount even if they did not have occasion to use any health services. This was called a *community rate*. Whatever the cost was for providing hospital care for everyone in the community (i.e., everyone who signed on for the insurance plan in the region it was operating), plus administrative expenses, determined the *premium* that the enrollees were charged for the coming year. Third, the plan was created by a hospital whose primary concern was covering its costs. Accordingly, Blue Cross paid whatever the hospital charged.

The Blue Cross plan was not designed to monitor hospital costs. Critics have pointed this out, noting that the nature of the plan permitted hospitals to spend as much as they wanted because they could be certain that their expenses would be covered. Blue Cross put no lid on expenditures. Defenders say, that is true, but there were important benefits in this arrangement. By shifting their costs to those who were insured, hospitals could provide care for people who could not afford to be hospitalized. *Cost shifting* became an item on the agenda of public debate during the 1980s. Critics said it was objectionable because it allowed hospitals to be irresponsible about their expenditures and it was unfair to the individuals who were insured but not being hospitalized.

There was nothing underhanded or secret about cost shifting. This was the accustomed method doctors and hospitals used before rates for health care services became standardized. Doctors charged richer patients more than they charged those who had less money. Everyone understood that this was happening. Doctors also accepted "payment in kind" from those who could not pay in cash, such as house repairs or other services. In practicing cost shifting, hospitals were just following an already well-established pattern. Critics point out that some patients received no care under these conditions if they could not find a doctor willing to treat them for no money.

When patterns of behavior are followed on a regular basis, sociologists say that the behavior patterns are being institutionalized. One particularly interesting effect of the institutionalized process in this case deserves a little more attention. Because Blue Cross would only pay for hospital care, and not care in the doctor's office, doctors would routinely admit patients to the hospital for tests. Doctors would explain the Blue Cross reimbursement arrangements to patients and ask if they would agree to have the necessary tests done in the hospital. The catch was that, officially, Blue Cross would only pay for hospitalization if the patient was sick. Acknowledging this reality, doctors routinely admitted patients with a diagnosis that proved to be negative after the appropriate tests were performed.

Consider the implications of this pattern of behavior. It is less expensive to have tests done on people who walk in, have the test done, and go home. It is much more expensive to keep people in the hospital. Also, as long as the person was going to be there anyway, doctors ordered more tests to justify admitting the person in the first place. Remember that Blue Cross was in the business of reimbursing hospitals for the costs they incurred, so hospitals had no reason to object to this pattern. The hospitals were fully aware of these practices. It was pretty obvious that there were a lot of healthy people being admitted. Doctors were doing it to save their patients money. Patients did not complain about the inconvenience because it did save them money. Both doctors and patients could convince themselves that this was a more efficient way of carrying out tests, that the tests would be more accurate because patients could be monitored before and after the tests, and so on. Eventually, however, health care costs did begin to climb and people did start to complain about it. Now, who is to blame for letting the situation get out of hand? I will leave the answer to that question for you to ponder.

Private, for-profit insurance companies, which sold life insurance, were fairly well established by the 1930s. They exhibited no interest in offering health insurance until BC–BS developed its plan. The private insurance companies became interested during the early 1940s because demand for health insurance rose rather dramatically around this time. That happened because wages were frozen during World War II and one of the only things that employers could offer to attract workers who were scarce during the wartime period was better benefits, particularly health insurance. Employers discovered that health insurance was particularly attractive to workers. Consider how fast the health insurance business grew—in 1940, only 9 percent of the population had hospital insurance; by 1950 the proportion had risen to 50 percent.[2]

Many of the new insurance plans developed during this period were sponsored by privately owned, well-established life insurance companies. The privately owned insurance companies differed from the BC–BS plans in two major ways. First, they operated as *profit-making* rather than *nonprofit* enterprises. Second, they reimbursed their enrollees rather than the hospitals in an *indemnity* arrangement (i.e., private insurance companies reimbursed the individual and not the hospital for the costs incurred, meaning the doctor and the hospital billed the patient directly). However, the private companies did not revise the payment schedule used by BC–BS. Like BC–BS, they simply paid out whatever hospitals charged. They made sure that they would make a profit by increasing the premium they charged each year, which BC–BS was doing as well, even if it did not do so to earn a profit. This worked until people started to complain about rising costs.

Insurance companies could have tried to hold down costs much earlier, but no one was pressing them to do that. The economy was booming and health care costs were not rising very fast since insurance plans were far more limited than they are now and few insurance plans covered outpatient care. As the market for health insurance started to become more competitive, the privately owned insurance companies did begin competing on the basis of price. They began setting premiums based on an "experience" or "risk rating" rather than using a "community rating." In other words, they calculated how often particular groups of customers went to the hospital and set the rate accordingly. Furthermore, they began aggressively recruiting customers who would be less likely to run up high health care costs. This has come to be known as "cherry picking" and "cream skimming."

It obviously doesn't take a rocket scientist to figure out that you can attract more business by reducing the premium you charge. The for-profit insurance companies began marketing their plans to organizations employing younger, healthier workers who had safe, quiet office jobs, and, of course, charging less for the offering. When this strategy was initially being developed companies were retiring their employees at the age of sixty-five. Insurance companies were not concerned about signing up people who sat all day, probably smoked, and did not get any exercise, because the chances were good that they would not suffer ill health until after they retired (often very shortly after they retired) and the company was no longer insuring them. So the private companies succeeded in attracting the younger, healthier employees who were less likely to go into the hospital by charging them less than the BC-BS plans. The BC-BS plans (now more commonly referred to as the "Blues") could not do the same thing because their legal status was that of nonprofit organizations (which meant that they did not have to pay taxes as long as they observed the conditions that made them nonprofits). Accordingly, the Blues could not tailor their rates to particular groups of people. They had to offer a community rate (the same rate for everyone), which was often higher than the experience rate or risk rate (which varied according to the characteristics of the group). Employers, who were becoming more interested in keeping their operating costs down, began offering the less expensive private insurance plans as an alternative to BC-BS.

How would you respond if you were heading up a Blues plan in your region? The only way you can compete with the private insurance companies is to employ the same business practices as they do. In order to offer competitive rates you would have to turn yourself into a profit-making corporation, exactly like the private insurance companies with whom you must compete. Not only did Blues plans turn themselves into for-profit plans, they consolidated their operations through mergers, acquisitions, and joint ventures with for-profit insurers. By 1999, the number of BC-BS plans had fallen from 128 at the peak of expansion to 51.[3] The trend did not let up until the middle of the first decade of the twenty-first century.

THE PREPAID CARE MODEL

It seems that after some small false starts here and there across the country, the idea of prepaid care took root in about 1938 in connection with the construction of the Los Angeles aqueduct. The area was unsettled, with primitive living conditions. Workers were willing to tolerate that, but they were not willing to do dangerous work without some assurance of medical care. No doctor would go to such a setting without some assurances of his own, namely that he could make enough money to set up an office and meet office and living expenses. Henry Kaiser, who headed the company doing the building, hit on a solution. He would guarantee the doctor a predictable income by arranging to have his workers contribute 5 cents per day to assure themselves of the availability of health care services whether they needed care or not. That worked so well that Kaiser set up similar programs for his employees during World War II to attract workers to jobs at his shipyards and steel mills in other locations on the West Coast. In 1942, he created a separate organization, Kaiser Permanente, to handle the prepaid health care arrangements for his workers.

When the war ended, wartime production declined, and employment shifted to other sectors, it looked like Kaiser Permanente would not survive. Henry Kaiser saved the plan by opening it up to the public. And, as they say, the rest is history. Kaiser Permanente evolved into the largest single prepaid care system in the country. As of 2011, it reports having 8.7 million enrollees and a $42.1 billion operating budget.

A few other prepaid plans, which stayed local, formed at about the same time as the Kaiser plan. The Health Insurance Plan of Greater New York and the Group Health Cooperative of Puget Sound were two of the largest. Prepaid care arrangements were relatively rare because there was so much opposition to them from the medical establishment (i.e., the AMA and its state and local affiliates). The fee-for-service exchange between the doctor and the patient was one of the traditional, and essential, attributes of medical professionalism according to the AMA. Accordingly, medical societies pressured hospitals to deny admitting privileges (i.e., the right to hospitalize patients) to doctors who were not in a fee-for-service practice. This forced the prepaid plans to build their own hospitals.

The plans that emerged during the first half of the twentieth century were established as nonprofit entities. The nonprofit aspect is significant. Remember, this means that there are no shareholders and no profits to distribute. If earnings exceed projected costs, the "excess" is plowed back into the organization.

FROM PREPAID CARE TO HEALTH MAINTENANCE

The prepaid care model got an enormous boost from legislation passed in 1974. At the time, President Richard Nixon was searching for a way to put limits on the growth of medical care costs once it had become apparent that the costs of Medicare and Medicaid (established in 1965) were running over initial cost projections. Advisors convinced President Nixon that prepaid care was the solution. Advocates argued that prepaid care would result in savings because the arrangement would encourage people to seek care earlier, before their problems became more complicated and costly to treat. So, not only was it going to save money, it would be good for people. President Nixon presented the plan to the country as something that would help people maintain their health, which is where the "health maintenance" label comes from. The medical establishment could not object to this presentation, even though it was firmly opposed to the prepayment feature. That did not stop the AMA from labeling it "socialized medicine" in a massive media campaign. The AMA's objections notwithstanding, legislation requiring employers to offer this option to their employees and funding to support startup costs passed and the term "health maintenance organization," or HMO, came into widespread use as of that time.

The way this model was designed to work was that both patients and doctors would sign up with a particular HMO. Doctors would do so by signing a contract. There was no restriction on doctors signing up with more than one HMO. The earliest HMOs paid doctors a salary; others offered doctors a contract specifying a fixed amount of money per capita—a *capitation fee*. As the HMO model developed, payment arrangements became more complicated. HMOs are now more likely to use capitation plus incentives for meeting the organization's budgetary objectives.

Patients would sign on by "enrolling" in a plan that employers had to agree to offer as a benefit option to employees. The employer would contract with the HMO to pay a fixed amount of money, the *premium*, to which the employee would contribute a set amount determined by the employer. Patients would be permitted to go only to those doctors who were associated with that particular HMO. HMOs continue to operate under this basic arrangement. Employers who were offering health insurance generally continued to offer the fee-for-service insurance option as well.

The fact that the legislation made a considerable amount of money available for startup costs brought many new parties into the prepaid care business, and business turns out to be the right word, too. Initially, the groups that took encouragement from the legislation used Kaiser Permanente as their model. They established themselves as nonprofit organizations. However, it did not take long for that to change. Within a few years, HMOs were being established with the understanding that producing a profit for their owners was exactly what the owners had in mind.

Many of the new HMOs, both for-profit and nonprofit, were established without enough planning, funding, or thought given to administration. Some of the struggling HMOs were bought out. Others simply closed up shop and disappeared. In either case, patients had to sign up with another, possibly new and untested organization, with new doctors, different rules, and so on. This is when the idea that the health care sector was inefficient, lacking in managerial talent, and backward in the application of the latest business techniques took hold. It is also when health sector corporations became more aggressive in their efforts to operate more efficiently in order to gain a greater share of the market, that is, more enrollees.

While the for-profit HMO may not have introduced business practices into the health care sector, it certainly accelerated the application of business practices. The newly evolving HMOs were interested in experimenting with a wide range of business management tools, most notably, software programs that monitor doctors' practice patterns. Collecting and analyzing such information permitted managed care organizations to press doctors to cut the number of patient visits, control the use of expensive tests, and generally reduce expenses associated with treatment.

Those who favored the expansion of the HMO approach interpreted this to mean that the most successful organizations were putting the less successful ones out of business because the successful ones were clearly offering a better product. While that might have been disruptive, having more effective and efficient organizations take over those that were not performing as well was justified as a temporary adjustment period that would work out just fine in the end. Isn't that the way it is supposed to work in this country?

It took a few more years for HMO executives to realize that one of the main obstacles they faced in trying to control costs or, more importantly, to make a profit, was that the HMOs could only control the costs of patient care taking place within the doctor's office. However, once patients were admitted to the hospital, the HMO lost control. HMOs did have contracts with hospitals covering basic costs per day, but could not really control the additional costs incurred once the patient was admitted. Thus, things like how long a patient was there, what tests were performed, how many times tests were repeated, which all have a big impact on costs, were not under the control of the HMO. They needed to gain more control over the hospital and thus over every other stage of care. That meant managing the care of the patient at all stages of treatment. This is what brought us to the next iteration in the labeling process—the era of *managed care*. Managing patient care led to managing the organizations and all the personnel patients interact with.

As HMOs became larger and more powerful, they were able to demand better deals in negotiations with hospitals and all the companies from which they order equipment and supplies (economies of scale). In many cases, managed care organizations could and ultimately did simply buy out their suppliers (vertical integration). This created even larger and more powerful organizations. Business executives argued that it was self-evident that "competition is healthy!" And that explains how we moved from the HMO label to the *managed competition* label. Managed competition was the foundational idea on which the Clinton health care reform plan was based. The managed competition concept was tainted by the failure of the Clinton health care reform proposal and fell into disfavor. Health insurance companies announced that they would prefer their offerings to be known as "health care plans."

As to personnel, HMOs had traditionally relied on generalists or primary care practitioners (PCPs), as opposed to specialists or surgeons, to a greater extent than is true outside of the HMO. The internists, pediatricians, and family practitioners, the PCPs, were expected to act as gatekeepers. They were, and still are, responsible for treating most of the patient's problems—referring patients to a specialist only if a problem truly required considerably more specialized knowledge. By monitoring the patient's care more closely, gatekeepers kept patients out of the hospital, which is beneficial to the patient (unless, of course, that effort becomes too restrictive). Hospitalization is the main form of care that HMOs intentionally tried to restrict because it is obviously so much more expensive than care provided in the doctor's office.

Curiously, even though employers had seen little evidence that managed care was reducing costs during the 1980s, they suddenly became convinced that managed care was the way to go during the 1990s. They began dropping traditional insurance as an alternative in the health care benefit packages they were offering to employees. In 1993, about half of American workers (versus the population as a whole) were enrolled in managed care programs; by 1995, that figure leaped to 73 percent).[4] The speed of the shift surprised everyone. While the pros and cons regarding the impact of managed care continued to mount, the number of people enrolled in health maintenance plans increased steadily through the decade of the 1990s. Enrollment peaked in 1999 at 30.1 million and has been declining ever since.[5] You might think that the rise in numbers of people enrolled in plans dedicated to the application of business practices would have brought more stable if not lower health insurance premiums. Not so! Annual premiums continued to rise, in fact, at double-digit percentage rates during a period when the rate of inflation was around 3 percent.

Enrollees continued to express dissatisfaction with the HMO model. While they were unhappy about the rising costs, they registered most dissatisfaction about the restrictions imposed by HMOs on which doctors they could see. This led to the introduction of a variation known as the "preferred provider organization," or PPO. The PPO option allowed enrollees to pay a higher premium for the right to select doctors of their own choosing. When that adjustment did not seem to fully overcome enrollee dissatisfaction, a "point-of-service" (POS) option appeared. This required the enrollee to select a primary care physician from the approved list who would assume responsibility for recommending a specialist if necessary. The POS was offered at a higher premium than the HMO premium, but one that was lower than the PPO option. Critics were quick to point out that the alternative arrangements were giving employers an excuse to revise benefit plans and pass on a greater proportion of the premium to employees.

Health plans took the opportunity to promote the PPO and POS as innovations rising out of the preferences consumers were registering, that is, presenting it all as the new era of "consumer-driven health care." One of the other options health plans have been promoting in recent years as part of the consumer-driven health care arrangements they are offering is the *high deductible plan* option. Such plans carry a lower premium because insurance coverage starts after the enrollee spends a substantial amount of money out of his or her own pocket; depending on the plan this could be $1,000, $2,000 or more. This is the deductible. (The plans are sometimes called catastrophic health insurance plans—get it? You really only get to use those benefits in case of a health catastrophe.) To make the high deductible option more attractive, legislation passed in 2003 creating health savings accounts (HSAs). The HSA allows the enrollee to set aside a certain amount of pretax income in a tax-free account to be used to cover medical costs that fall in the deductible range. (The HSA replaced an earlier version of this plan called the "flexible spending account," which was more restrictive.)

According to a 2008 study by the Government Accountability Office, the average income of those who opt for the HSA plan is $139,000 compared to the income of average enrollees, which is $57,000. In short, there are those who say that this is another tax loophole that serves the rich and is not something that benefits most Americans.

That brings us to a rather basic question, namely, whether the HMO approach to health care delivery is bringing us larger, more efficient health care networks that are beneficial to patients and to society as a whole. Some argue that the business approach employed by health insurance companies brought greater efficiency and greater responsiveness to consumer preference, and that market competition is the only way to control rising costs. The reality is that the primary objective of for-profit health plans is making money. It is their "legal, ethical, and fiduciary responsibility" to do so.[6] Most observers agree that nonprofit HMOs have had to operate by the same rules in order to survive. Accordingly, the industry as a whole refers to the money spent on medical care as the "medical-*loss* ratio." The money spent on medical care carries a negative label because of its negative impact on the bottom line. The logic that flows from the use of that concept is obvious—cut medical care services in order to increase profits.

Critics say that consolidation is less a matter of efficiency than an attempt to increase control over the market. And that brought us health care monopolies that are more interested in shareholder benefits than health benefits to enrollees. Consider the fact that five of the biggest health plans in the country enrolled 68 million persons in 2003, that is about 89 percent of all HMO enrollees, given that the total enrollment was about 76 million or so that year.[7]

The five top HMOs got to where they are because of numerous previous mergers. This is when the Federal Trade Commission (FTC) and states' attorneys started to take an interest, because the number of insurers had clearly been declining. The FTC's concern was that certain mergers would produce organizations so large that their size would result in restraint of trade, that is, that they would be the major and perhaps only insurer in the area. States' attorneys were concerned that the enrollees in their states would get less attention from bigger and more powerful plans. Policy makers and, more to the point, the courts were weighing this question: are health plan mergers helping to contain costs or does consolidation of such magnitude create monopolies with the power to set prices for the purpose of enhancing profit with no real interest in containing costs?

The AMA is certain that absence of competition in the health insurance market puts both doctors and patients at a disadvantage. According to a 2011 AMA assessment of the health insurance market, 99 percent of health insurance markets in the United States are "highly concentrated," based on the 1997 U.S. Department of Justice and Federal Trade Commission Horizontal Merger Guidelines. This indicates a significant absence of competition among insurers. In 48 percent of metropolitan statistical areas, at least one insurer had a market share of 50 percent or more.[8]

Another criticism of health insurance companies that surfaces periodically revolves around the compensation awarded to company executives. This criticism was for some reason heard more often during the middle of the first decade of the twenty-first century than it has been over the last few years, probably because attention has switched rather decisively to debates about the pros and cons of health care reform. Critics were more apt to point out then that the health plan executives were getting rich by denying care to people who are sick. A case in point was the 2003 package that went to Aetna's CEO, John Rowe.[9] He received $1,042,146 in salary, a $2.2 million bonus, new stock options that were estimated to be worth $5.6 million, and a $7 million cash payment on stock options, plus other compensation of nearly $400,000. That is a staggering $16,242,146 in total. Other officers of the company received huge compensation packages as well that year. One group of investors decided to take action. The United Association of Plumbers, Pipefitters & Sprinklerfitters proposed to shareholders and the board of directors of Aetna that Rowe's compensation package be limited to $1 million and annual bonuses be linked to performance measures. The board rejected the proposal saying that it was too rigid. The union's move was undoubtedly spurred on by the company's decision to fire 10,700 employees and lay off an additional 700 over the previous year.

Over the last few years, attention seems to have shifted away from the compensation going to health insurance company CEOs, if not CEOs of other companies. Rising stock values and the reasons behind this trend are now attracting greater attention. According to one report, "Profits at the nation's seven largest publicly traded insurers went up in 2010 as plans spent less on care and used income to buy back their stock to boost per-share earnings."[10]

There are also those who point out that health insurance companies are making a modest profit compared to some other industries. Some estimates put profits at 3 to 4 percent. This is in contrast to what the business pages will tell you is the most profitable industry in the United States, that is, mining and crude oil extraction, which reported just under 20 percent in annual profits in 2009. More closely related to this discussion, would you be surprised to discover that the pharmaceutical industry is the second most profitable industry, reporting a return of 19.8 percent in 2009? How much profit is reasonable when we are dealing with people's pain and suffering and medications that might help as well as medications that people don't really need but are being convinced will perform miracles by the constant barrage of ads? I will let you come up with an answer for that question.

Coverage and Cost of Workplace Health Insurance

Let's first take a closer look at how many people receive health insurance through their employers and then consider the plight of those who are not receiving this benefit. As costs began to escalate, employers initially tried to cut their costs by switching to less expensive plans and limiting the number of plans employees could choose from. However, this did little to cap the steady rise in costs. Over time, employers began dropping the health insurance benefit. In 1984, 69.1 percent of Americans got their health insurance through their employer; by 2009, the percentage had dropped to 58 percent.[11]

By now you might be wondering how expensive health insurance really is. Let's look at how much it costs employers to offer insurance, and employees to sign on to a health insurance plan. The following is based on a Kaiser Family Foundation survey. The percentage of firms offering health insurance increased to 69 percent in 2010, largely due to an increase in offering among firms with three to nine workers. In other words, even though an increasing number of companies have started to offer insurance, larger companies with more employees were dropping insurance coverage, so that fewer people were being covered by insurance. The average premium in 2010 was $5,049 for single coverage and $13,770 for family coverage. There has been a significant increase in cost since 2000. In 2000, the employee portion was $1,619; the employer's portion was $4,819 for a total of $6,438. The difference between employer-sponsored insurance in 2000 and 2010 amounts to a 114 percent rise in total cost but a much bigger increase at 147 percent in the worker's share of costs. The 2010 cost to the employer for family coverage is $9,773 and $3,997 to the employee.[12] Doesn't that go a long way in explaining why so many people have been saying that something has to be done about the cost of health care services?

Insurance companies are well aware of the fact that about 5 percent of enrollees run up most of the costs. Knowing this, they calculate the risks posed by the population they are selling insurance to, that is, a particular company's employees, and set the rates accordingly. Enrolling individuals is much riskier, especially individuals who have had previous health problems. Enrolling such people is a risk that just does not make sense from the perspective of insurance companies. Why accept such risk if you don't have to? Insurance companies have never been under any obligation to provide health insurance to everyone who applies for it. That will change as a result of the health care reform act.

The Individual Health Insurance Market

That brings us to the question of what one can do if one's employer decides to drop health insurance as a benefit, or if one is self-employed, or works for a small company that has never offered health insurance benefits. Why can't one just go out and buy an individual health insurance policy, recognizing that it will be somewhat more expensive than getting insurance through employment?

A small proportion of the population does obtain health insurance on their own in what is known as the individual health insurance market. In 2009, 5.3 percent of the population bought their own health insurance.[13] Why then aren't more people buying their own health insurance as employers cut back on this benefit? There are two basic reasons. One, they can't afford it, and two, insurance companies will not sell it to them. Consider the story told by a woman whose husband is retired and who found herself without insurance when her company was bought out and she lost her job.

> My husband, teenage daughter and I were all active and healthy, and naively thought getting health insurance would be simple. . . . First, we wanted to know that, if we had a medical catastrophe, we would not

exhaust our savings. Second, uninsured patients are billed more than the rates that insurers negotiate with doctors and hospitals, and we wanted to pay those lower rates. The difference is significant: my recent MRI cost $1,300 at the "retail" rate, while the rate negotiated by the insurance company was $700. . . . (in filling out the application) I diligently listed the various minor complaints for which we had been seen over the years, knowing that these might turn up later and be a basis for revoking coverage if they were not disclosed.

Then the first letter arrived—denied. . . . Why were we denied? What were these preexisting conditions that put us into high-risk categories? For me, it was a corn on my toe for which my podiatrist had recommended an in-office procedure. My daughter was denied because she takes a regular medication for a common teenage issue. My husband was denied because his ophthalmologist had identified a slow-growing cataract. . . .

I completed four applications for each of the three of us, using reams of paper. I learned to read the questions carefully. I mulled over the difference between a "condition" and "something for which you have sought treatment." I was precise and succinct. I felt as if was doing a deposition.[14]

She goes on to say that she was not able to obtain a family policy but was able to obtain individual health insurance policies for each of them. Their individual premiums increased substantially over the last six years with an average increase of 20 percent per year. What is important to realize about this story is how many people are in the same situation.

The economic recession that we experienced over the last few years of the first decade of the twenty-first century caused the ranks of the unemployed to swell. A study carried out by the Commonwealth Fund found that of the 3,033 persons surveyed nearly one-quarter lost their jobs between 2008 and 2010. That is about 43 million people. "Of the estimated 26 million adults who bought, or tried to buy, health insurance on the individual insurance market in the past three years, 16 million found it very difficult or impossible to find a plan they could afford. An estimated 9 million were turned down or charged a higher price because of a health problem, or a preexisting condition that excluded them from their coverage."[15]

Okay, so you can't get insurance. How about paying for health care services when you need them until you get a job and have insurance again through employment? Part of the problem is that as an individual you have no bargaining power. Most of us would go to the hospital and have an essential or life-saving surgical procedure done without weighing the costs and benefits, right? Then you get the bill. Your bill will be a lot higher than the bill insured people receive for the same procedure because the insurance company has entered into a contract with the hospital on how much the hospital will charge. As someone without insurance coverage you will be charged the non-negotiated amount. Can you negotiate after the fact? Maybe. Will you be able to afford the renegotiated charge—maybe, maybe not. And, that explains why so many people are going into medical bankruptcy.

Legislation has been in place since 1986 requiring insurance companies to provide continued coverage for a certain period of time after the employee leaves his or her place of employment. This is known as COBRA (passed under the Consolidated Omnibus Budget Reconciliation Act of 1986). The legislation does not address costs. Insurance companies can charge whatever they want for continued coverage. As a result, a person who is suddenly un-employed might not be able to pay for individual coverage even though he or she is entitled to receive that coverage.

Now that you understand how health insurance works—it's about to change. We will now consider how the Affordable Care Act will change health insurance as we know it.

HEALTH CARE REFORM—THE INDIVIDUAL MANDATE

The *individual mandate* is one of the most controversial parts of the health care reform law. The law requires every individual in the country, with some very clearly outlined exceptions, to have health insurance as of 2014. Those who do not obtain coverage will have to pay an annual fine. The amount of the fine will be phased in: $95 in 2014 or 1 percent of taxable income; $325 in 2015 or 2 percent of taxable income; $695 per person or 2.5 percent of tax-able income up to a maximum of $2,085 per family income as of 2016. After 2016, the fine will be increased annually by the cost-of-living adjustment. Exceptions are allowed for a limited number of reasons, including financial hardship, religious objections, for those without coverage for less than three months, incarcerated persons, undocumented immigrants, and American In-dians. An exception will also be made for those whose incomes fall below the tax filing threshold and those who are unable to find a plan that costs less than 8 percent of the person's income. Individuals whose incomes fall below 133 percent of the federal poverty level will be eligible for Medicaid coverage as of 2014. (We will discuss government-sponsored, public programs including Medicaid in the following chapter.)

The rationale for requiring all individuals to purchase health insurance is that it prevents people from buying insurance only when they need it. As some pundits put it, deciding to buy it on the way to the hospital. Having healthy people as well as sick people in the insurance pool spreads the risk. As you will recall this is the basis on which Blue Cross was founded. To ensure that individuals have a range of insurance plans from which to choose, states are being mandated to establish *Health Benefit Exchanges*. Funding is being made available to states to establish the exchanges which must be fully functioning by 2014. The U.S. Office of Personnel Management is required to contract with insurers to offer at least two multi-state plans in each exchange. At least one of the plans must be offered by a nonprofit entity and at least one plan must exclude coverage for abortions.

The Health Benefit Exchange

Insurers must meet certain qualifications to participate in the exchanges. They must have adequate provider networks, be accredited, perform well with respect to quality measures, and so on. They must agree to report information on claims payments, enrollment and disenrollment, number of claims denied, cost-sharing, and so on. Insurance companies will be allowed to "risk rate," that is, charge some people more, on the basis of age, but no more than three times more from youngest to oldest enrollees.

The feature that people shopping for health insurance are likely to appreciate most is the requirement that insurance companies state what they will cover in plain language so that potential enrollees can compare plans to one another using the same criteria. Won't that be interesting? Other rules that enrollees will appreciate include the following: insurers will be prohibited from imposing lifetime limits on coverage; will be prohibited from rescinding coverage except in cases of fraud; will have to present plans to increase premiums for review; waiting periods for coverage will be limited to ninety days; young adults will be able to stay on their parents' health plans until age twenty-six.

Health insurance plans will have to fall into one of four benefit categories that specify responsibility for *out-of-pocket* costs plus one catastrophic category.

The four categories are as follows:

- Bronze plan—provides basic coverage; those who purchase this plan will be responsible for paying for 40 percent of costs out of their own pockets (there are going to be out-of-pocket limits linked to income as outlined below)
- Silver plan—provides basic coverage with 30 percent out-of-pocket costs
- Gold plan—enrollees with have to pay 20 percent out-of-pocket
- Platinum plan—enrollees will pay 10 percent out-of-pocket
- Catastrophic plan—available to persons 30 years and under; three primary care visits are covered; all else is out of pocket and the prevailing out-of-pocket limit applies.

Out-of-pocket expenses are tied to percentage of the federal poverty level up to 400 percent of poverty. Individuals earning between 100 and 200 percent of poverty will not be expected to pay more than $1,983 out of pocket. Those earning between 300 and 400 percent of poverty will have a ceiling of $3,987 in out-of-pocket expenditures. Premium subsidies will also be available to families with incomes up to 400 percent of poverty. Based on 2009 calculations, families will receive a subsidy of $29,327 to $88,200 for a family of four.

Because the exchanges, with a couple of exceptions, do not exist, a number of important issues will have to be worked out. One such issue is the question of whether insurance agents will be involved. If people will be buying insurance through agents, that will raise the cost of the insurance. Agents have typically charged a 15 to 20 percent fee. If people will be buying directly from the exchanges, will the process and information be clear enough that people will be comfortable doing so without the help of an agent? We shall have to watch and see how this question gets settled.

Changes to Private Insurance Plans

Health insurance plans were required to report the proportion of premium dollars they spend on clinical services, quality, and other costs as of 2010 when the health care reform act was signed. Furthermore, those that spent less than 85 percent on services to their enrollees were mandated to provide rebates to enrollees as of January 1, 2011. The remaining 15 percent, which we discussed earlier in connection with how much profit insurance companies are earning, is the *medical loss ratio*. This feature of the legislation effectively prohibits insurance plans from spending more than 15 percent on anything other than health care services, that is, administration, salaries, benefits, and distribution of profits. In the individual and small group market, the medical-loss ratio cap has been set at 20 percent.

A number of other restrictions will go into effect as of 2014. Some of the most important changes include limiting deductibles in the small group market to $2,000 for individuals and $4,000 for families, limiting waiting periods to 90 days, and prohibiting lifetime limits.

HEALTH CARE REFORM—EMPLOYER REQUIREMENTS

The law requires employers with two hundred employees to enroll them in a plan selected by the employer. The legislation will have little effect on large companies that have been providing health insurance for their employees all along. The law allows employees to opt out of employer coverage and seek individual coverage. The second most controversial part of the legislation, after the individual mandate, affects small employers. The rules that affect small employers are as follows:

- Employers who employ fifty or more people will be assessed a fee of $2,000 per full-time employee if they do not offer coverage and if they have at least one employee who receives a credit through a Health Insurance Exchange.
- Employers that offer coverage will be required to provide a voucher to employees whose incomes are below 400 percent of poverty if their share of the cost is 8 to 9 percent of their income.

Employers who employ twenty-five to fifty people whose annual wages average out to be less than $50,000 will receive a tax credit for providing health insurance to their employees. The rules on credit are as follows:

- If the employer contributes at least 50 percent of the cost of insurance, the employer will receive a tax credit of up to 35 percent of the contribution.
- Businesses with up to one hundred employees will be able to purchase insurance through Health Insurance Exchanges.
- As of 2017, states will have to have Small Business Health Options Program Exchanges in place where businesses with over one hundred employees will be able to purchase coverage.

Small employers who employ ten or fewer employees whose annual wages average out to $25,000 or less will be eligible for a full tax credit.

THE AMERICAN HEALTH
BENEFIT EXCHANGE—WILL IT WORK?

Two states, Massachusetts and Utah, have had such exchanges for a while.[16] In Massachusetts people file applications for subsidized coverage which they can obtain from one of five state-approved insurers. Massachusetts serves as the purchaser. It solicits bids from insurance companies and bargains over prices and benefits. In Utah, people go to a web site and sign up. Utah allows people to select from plans sold by any insurers who want to participate. The state defines the minimum benefits that insurers must offer, but after that steps back. The difference between the two approaches is clear. In one case, the state believes its citizens will get a better deal if the state limits competition to qualified vendors. In the other case, the state believes that relying on market forces will produce a better deal. Which approach other states choose to take is difficult to predict.

Exchanges are receiving so much close scrutiny for a couple of reasons. First, if a state does not have an exchange in place by 2014, the federal government will come in and set one up. Second, the law requires members of Congress to obtain their health insurance through the exchange—so they have reason to be interested in how the exchanges function.

How does the business community feel about the exchanges? It seems that small employers are generally pleased to have greater access to health insurance. Small businesses have been facing some of the same challenges that individuals have been facing in seeking insurance because a small pool is riskier to insure than a large pool of enrollees. Accordingly, the exchanges come as a relief to small businesses. Middle-sized companies are anticipating savings because the government will provide financial support for providing insurance. Large companies are not being affected, but might find less expensive plans through the exchanges. On the whole, business should benefit. And to the extent that the cost of health insurance is being passed on to employees in the form of reduced wages currently, employees may benefit as well when they are able to purchase health insurance at a lower cost.

If so many parties are likely to see economic benefit from health care reform, why is there is so much opposition? The answer at this point is that people's economic interests and political interests are not necessarily aligned. We will get back to this point in chapter 7 when we focus on public reaction to the law.

· *6* ·

Public Health Insurance

$\mathcal{T}$he federal government created three government-sponsored, that is, public, health insurance programs during the last half century: Medicare, the program for the elderly; Medicaid, the program for the poor; and the State Children's Health Insurance Program (CHIP) for low-income children. The government also operates programs that provide health care services for some other clearly specified categories of persons. This includes the Veterans Administration (VA) for veterans, the Indian Health Service for Native Americans, and military hospitals and clinics for active military service personnel.

Medicare and social security are considered "entitlement" programs, that is, benefit programs that people are entitled to because they have earned those benefits over their lifetime by working and contributing to these programs. This is in contrast to programs for which people qualify because they don't have the "means" to purchase the services they need—these are known as "means tested" programs. Medicaid and CHIP are means-tested programs.

The programs are complicated. I leave it to you to decide whether they are more complicated than the private insurance plans we have just looked at. If you end up feeling overwhelmed by how much you need to know about the plans, just imagine how the people who try to enroll in these plans must feel, especially the elderly, who may not be so comfortable with obtaining information found on Internet sites.

MEDICARE

The Medicare program was legislated in 1965 as an amendment (Title 18) to the Social Security Act. It went into operation in July of 1966; the first full year of operation was 1967. It was designed to provide health insurance for people over the age of sixty-five. As you will recall from an earlier discussion, this was done because the elderly were identified as particularly vulnerable. They were found to be at greater risk of not having the resources to pay for health care and at greater risk of experiencing illness. The focus on poverty in the early 1960s led to the discovery that an unexpectedly high proportion of older Americans were poor. Making things more complicated, not only were poor Americans unable to afford to buy their own health insurance after retirement, it was not readily available on an individual basis, especially not to people over the age of sixty-five.

Most Americans become eligible for Medicare once they reach the age of sixty-five. Younger persons who are permanently disabled or blind may qualify as well. Persons with end-stage renal disease (meaning it is fatal unless the person has a kidney transplant) were included in 1972 because someone in Congress advocated for it and no one particularly objected.

The plan is complex. The following describes the plan before the changes outlined in the ACA reform act go into effect. Medicare was originally established as a two-part program: Part A is the hospital insurance portion and Part B covers physicians' fees. Two newer parts, labeled Parts C and D, were added later. Part C, which is now known as Medicare-Advantage, is an option that allows people to join Medicare-approved, alternative plans offered by private insurance companies that combine Parts A and B and sometimes include Part D. Part D is the prescription drug plan legislated in 2003.

Anyone who receives social security or Railroad Retirement Board benefits is automatically eligible for Part A. Persons who did not pay in to the Social Security Fund through employment are not eligible. Part B covers doctors' services, is voluntary, and carries a monthly charge, which is deducted from the person's monthly social security check. A person must sign up for each of these benefit programs once the person is eligible—for social security and for both Parts A and B of Medicare. Medicare enrollees may choose to purchase C and D plans from private insurance companies. The government outlines all the components of the Medicare plan in a manual that is updated every year and sent out to all enrollees and made available on its web site as well.

As of 2010 Medicare enrolled 47.5 million persons. It had an income of $486 billion and expenditures of $523 billion. That makes it the most expensive of the three public health programs but not the largest in terms of enrollment. These figures also raise concerns about sustainability, which we will address later in this discussion.

That brings us to funding. Part A is funded through a 1.45 percent deduction from an employee's check plus a 1.45 percent contribution on the part of the employer. Part A operates as follows: enrollees must pay coinsurance for each hospitalization during each "spell of illness." In 2011, this amounted to a total of $1,132 for each hospital stay of 1 to 60 days during the year; $283 per day for days 61–90; $566 per day for days 91–150; and the total cost for each day beyond 150. There is a lifetime reserve of 60 days which can be used only once over a person's lifetime.

Part A also covers skilled nursing home care, but sets strict limitations. Coverage is available for one hundred days, but only if the person is admitted after three or more days of hospitalization. There is no coinsurance for the first twenty days. As of the twenty-first day, there is a charge of up to $141.50 per day. After one hundred days, Medicare pays nothing. Home health care and hospice care are covered, again under strict limitations.

Part B is funded through a deduction in the enrollee's social security check, if and when the person signs up for it. Until recently, everyone paid the same amount. As of 2011 the amount is linked to income level. The deduction for persons whose income is under $85,000 per year is $115.40 per month. There are five income levels. For those in the highest income level, that is, over $214,000, the monthly deduction is $369.10. In addition to the monthly premium, enrollees pay a deductible of $162 once per calendar year and 20 percent of all Medicare-approved doctor and outpatient charges. Part B also covers durable medical equipment (e.g., rental of a hospital-type bed) and certain nondurables (e.g., dialysis supplies). Laboratory tests are usually fully covered.

The Medicare plan does not cover a number of things that you might expect it to cover, like long-term nursing home care after one hundred days, which we just mentioned. Since there are a lot of people in nursing homes—who is paying for their care? It turns out that Medicaid is probably paying. We will get back to that. Medicare does not pay for dental care, hearing aids, and hearing exams, routine eye care and most eyeglasses, or such necessities as adult diapers.

Because coinsurance and deductibles can run into a lot of money, Medigap insurance was created. There are fourteen standardized Medigap plans; they can be sold by any private insurance company that wishes to offer any of them, as long as the plan covers whatever is specified in plans identified by the letters A through N. The government publishes a booklet in hard-copy and online versions outlining what the plans identified by each letter are supposed to cover. Companies are permitted to set the prices they charge and claim that they provide better administrative services. They cannot claim that they will provide more health care services than specified by the plan under that letter. That certainly makes it easier for Medicare enrollees to determine which Medigap policy to buy based on what they can afford and what they want covered. There is far less chance of confusion than there has been to date about what is covered because the government has eliminated what we think of as the "fine print."

Part C was known as Medicare + Choice when it was introduced in 1997. Under this arrangement, Medicare was to pay private insurance companies a fixed fee to provide a package of health care services, combining Parts A and B. The number of plans grew to 345 by the following year. When the government looked into who was choosing to enroll in Medicare + Choice plans, it discovered that enrollees were generally younger and healthier than the general Medicare population. Moreover, it found that those who did become seriously ill proceeded to drop out of these plans and shift back to the traditional Medicare plan. Given these findings, Medicare determined that it was overpaying and proceeded to reduce the rate that it was offering private insurance companies to provide alternative plans. Medicare + Choice plans responded by increasing their out-of-pocket charges. By 1999, 17 percent of the Medicare eligible population opted for this alternative. The out-of-pocket charges averaged $429 that year. The charges rose steadily after that. By 2003 charges stood at $1,260 per year. By 2004 the number of plans had dropped to 145 and the number of enrollees had dropped to 11 percent.[1]

The rules governing Medicare + Choice were revised in 2003 in conjunction with the passage of Part D, the Medicare Prescription Drug, Improvement, and Modernization Act. The Part C part of the plan was renamed Medicare Advantage. In passing this legislation the government agreed to pay insurance companies 8.4 percent more per Medicare Advantage enrollee than for enrollees in the Part A and B traditional plan. Proponents presented it as a cost containment measure. The members of Congress who presented this argument said that private companies needed an incentive to offer alternatives to government plans, which would ultimately reduce costs through competition because private companies were sure to introduce cost-saving innovation. By all accounts, over the next few years the amount the government was paying private companies over and above the cost of Part A and Part B edged up to 14 percent, reaching a high of 19 percent some in rural areas.[2]

Those who opt for Medicare Advantage coverage in 2011 may choose from an average of twenty-four plans offered by insurance companies in each respective community, some of which may include a cap on out-of-pocket expenses.[3] About half of the plans available in 2010 included a $3,400 cap. Nearly 80 percent include drug coverage but generally not comprehensive drug coverage. About a quarter of Medicare beneficiaries were enrolled in Medicare Advantage plans as of 2011.

That brings us to Part D, the prescription drug legislation, the Medicare Prescription Drug, Improvement, and Modernization Act, signed into law in

2003 at a cost of $395 billion. Two months later, the White House announced that it had recalculated that figure and found that it would actually cost $534 billion.[4] Unfortunately, this came at a time when the costs of the war in Iraq were running higher than predicted and the economy was not improving as fast as the White House had said it would.

Part D went into effect in 2006. Part D was designed to be offered by private insurance companies. Medicare enrollees could select from a range of plans offered by private companies and sign up on a voluntary basis. The unique feature of the plan, the doughnut hole, was the result of the compromise that Congress reached because there was not enough money to provide for full coverage. It operates as follows: in the first year of operation, the plan covered 75 percent of drug costs up to $2,250. After that, the person would pay 100 percent for drugs—putting the person in the doughnut hole. After a person spent $5,100, coverage would kick back in again to cover 95 percent of the cost of drugs. Expenditures between $2,250 and $5,100 defined the doughnut hole. The doughnut hole was scheduled to change in size with every passing year as was the percentage of costs covered beyond the doughnut hole. By 2011, enrollees were covered at the rate of 75 percent for expenditures up to $2,840; zero until $6,448, when coverage at the rate of 80 percent kicked in again.

Part D plans are sold by insurance companies on a state-by-state basis. The number of plans enrollees may choose from average around thirty or thirty-five per state. As of 2010, plans were being sold at a range of premiums from a low of $14.80 per month to a high of around $45.00. The rules for which drugs are covered and at what rate are complicated depending on whether the drugs are generic formulations and on a variety of other rules over which the government has little say.

Administration and Assessment of Success

The Medicare program is administered by the Centers for Medicare and Medicaid Services (CMS), which as you already know is a part of the Department of Health and Human Services. CMS does not employ staff to process Medicare claims. It enters into contracts with "carriers" who compete for the contracts. Health insurance companies (both nonprofit and for-profit) are called carriers when they agree to "carry out" the day-to-day administration of the program and earn a profit for doing so. The insurance companies do the paperwork and pay the bills submitted by hospitals and doctors who provide the health care services.

CMS also monitors the quality of the care for which it is paying. It requires that hospitals be accredited by the Joint Commission on Accreditation of Healthcare Organizations (JCAHO) which is the organization that reviews the performance of hospitals in the United States. CMS does its own reviews as well. It monitors doctors' performance by contracting with peer review organizations (PROs). Doctors perform the peer review, the idea being that you need to be a doctor to evaluate whether other doctors are doing a good job. PROs employ a staff of workers, usually nurses, who review Medicare files for the purpose of finding unusual patterns of treatment or charges. When there is some question about treatment, doctors who work with the PRO become involved.

Now that you see how the Medicare program is set up, the question that you might want to ask is: how well is it working? The answer depends on what you want it to accomplish. Obviously, Medicare cannot keep people from dying, nor can it keep people from aging and developing chronic illnesses. Most analysts agree that the Medicare program plays a major role in extending and improving the lives of enrollees.

The debate about how well Medicare is working largely revolves around how much it costs. The following facts should help explain why cost is such a big source of concern. To begin with, Medicare has been outpacing economic growth for many years, increasing at the rate of 7 percent per year in 1970 to 18 percent in 2009; and projected to reach 20 percent by 2020.

By 2008, one out of every five dollars spent on health care services was a Medicare dollar. Based on CMS calculations, by 2030 the program will enroll double the number of people who were enrolled in 2000. Spending on average is substantially higher for the oldest enrollees, who will be increasing in number over this time period. In 2006, the expenditure for beneficiaries ages sixty-five to seventy-four amounted to $5,887 per year; for those over eighty-five, it was $12,059 per year. Also, clear evidence shows that only a small proportion of enrollees account for the majority of expenditures. In 2006, spending for those in the top 10 percent of the Medicare expenditures averaged $48,210 in contrast to those in the bottom 90 percent for whom the average cost of coverage was $3,910.

The fact that the baby boom generation is entering its golden years as of 2011 explains why expenditure projections have been attracting the attention of policy experts and politicians who must sign off on funding. Consider these two facts: 1) about 76 million people were born between 1946 and 1964; 2) the fastest growing age group in the population is the over-eighty-five group.[5]

The Great Recession is presenting another source of worry. When the ACA was legislated, the Medicare Board of Trustees announced that the Trust Fund would extend the solvency of the Medicare Program by twelve years, moving it forward from 2017 to 2029. When the trustees reviewed that projection a year later, they concluded that Medicare will start running out of money as of 2024.[6] They attributed the change to the downturn in the economy.

After hearing why policy makers are so concerned about costs, we should stop to note an important positive observation about the way the program operates—it carries out its administrative responsibilities at a cost of 2 percent of program expenditures. On the not-so-positive side, Medicare fraud is growing into a vast industry that is very difficult to control. Now that the outlines of the Medicare program are clear—both its strengths and its weaknesses— the question is what impact will health care reform have on the Medicare Program?

MEDICARE AND HEALTH CARE REFORM

The reform law introduced a large number of changes, some quite broad and some very specific. The following presents an overview of the changes.

Some of the broad changes include the creation of a new Independent Payment Advisory Board charged with finding ways to reduce Medicare spending if spending exceeds the targeted growth rate. A number of new rules have been introduced aimed at preventing fraud, such as requiring providers to have face-to-face encounters with patients before certifying the need for home health services and requiring providers to be prepared to provide documentation upon request. Another anti-fraud mechanism is the creation of a database designed to document information on fraudulent activities that can be shared by federal and state programs. Changes that are specific to the four parts of the program include the following.

Part A: The payroll tax on higher income earners, individuals earning more than $200,000 and couples earning more than $250,000, will increase to 2.35 percent to be taken out of their paychecks instead of 1.45 percent; this is what everyone has been paying and everyone who earns less than the specified amounts will continue to pay.

Part B: Income related premiums have been frozen at the level set in 2010 and are not scheduled to increase until 2019.

Part C: The changes to Medicare Advantage are extensive:

- Plans will have to maintain an 85 percent medical-loss ratio. That means that insurance companies offering these plans will have to spend 85 percent on services, leaving 15 percent for profit and administration. If a plan exceeds this ratio for two years, Medicare will terminate the contract.

- Payment for services will be set using average Medicare costs by county, which will serve as benchmarks. Plans operating in the most costly counties will receive 95 percent of the county benchmark; those in lowest-cost counties will receive 115 percent. Benchmark payments will be phased in over a three-year period.
- Plans will be rated for quality using a five-star rating system established the year before the law was passed. Plans receiving a rating of four or more will receive bonus payments starting in 2012, which will increase over following years.
- A number of other changes will be introduced to take into account higher cost patients with chronic illness using a risk score formula.

Part D: Significant changes are being made to the drug benefit section of Medicare:

- All enrollees whose drug costs fell into the doughnut hole received a $250 rebate in the fall of 2010.
- Enrollees whose drug costs fall into the doughnut hole as of 2011 will receive a 50 percent discount on brand-name drugs and a reduction in coinsurance on generic drugs.
- The doughnut hole is gradually being reduced, meaning that by 2020 enrollees will pay 25 percent coinsurance for drugs rather than 100 percent once their expenditures hit the doughnut hole.
- Subsidies for low-income beneficiaries are being introduced and some payment arrangements that apply to the Indian Health Service are being altered.

The law also introduces changes in how it pays doctors and how much it pays them. For example, reimbursement to primary care physicians is being increased; annual wellness and prevention visits will be covered, which was not the case until now. It means that physicians will be reimbursed for such visits. Physicians practicing in health professional shortage areas will be paid 10 percent more than those in non-shortage areas. A pilot program is going into effect as of 2013 aimed at bundling services for an episode of care starting at the acute stage when the patient enters the hospital through the outpatient stage. The aim is to deliver care in a more coordinated way that would produce cost savings. Finally, physicians are banned from establishing new specialty hospitals in which they have a financial interest because they typically refer less risky patients to these hospitals. Thus the other hospitals with which they are affiliated, that offer comprehensive care, end up getting the patients who are sicker and more costly to treat. Multispecialty hospitals made it clear that they wanted the government to do something about the specialty hospitals.

MEDICAID

The other major public program, legislated at the same time as Medicare as an amendment (Title 19) to the Social Security Act, was Medicaid. Its first full year of operation was also 1967. Medicaid is a joint federal-state program created to provide health care services for particular categories of low-income people. They can be classified into three groupings: the poor elderly, people with disabilities who are too disabled to work, and poor single parents, generally women, with small children. Able-bodied adults, male and female, with no small children, no matter how poor, were ineligible.

The federal government allowed states a fair amount of leeway in determining eligibility. States were permitted to set the eligibility cutoff at a percent of the poverty level established by the federal government for the year, at 100 percent of poverty or well above or below that figure. The federal government picks up half of each state's Medicaid outlay, more if the state has an especially high proportion of poor people. This averages out to 57 percent of Medicaid costs across the states. Congress has also periodically enacted new requirements linked to expanded federal support. By 2003 the federal government had legislated a series of changes to the original law requiring states to provide coverage for twenty-eight additional specific categories of people and allowed states to cover up to twenty-one optional eligibility groups.[7] For example, the federal government began requiring coverage for children under age six and pregnant women at 133 percent of poverty. Coverage for children under age eighteen who were at 100 percent of poverty was also mandated. States were permitted to cover both parents and children in low-income families if they chose to do so.

The Medicaid program has experienced tremendous expansion and is now the largest of the three public programs with an enrollment of 58.2 million persons as of 2008. It costs the government $45.2 billion to operate. (Remember the Medicare program enrolls 45.2 million persons and costs $468.1 billion.) Table 6.1 outlines who is enrolled in the program and how enrollment has grown.

While all beneficiaries are entitled to health care services, they do not necessarily all seek health care. So it is important to look at who is receiving Medicaid services. Table 6.2 shows how Medicaid payments are distributed.

Table 6.1.   U.S. Medicaid Enrollees, 1972, 2000, and 2008

	*1972**	*2000*	*2008*
All beneficiaries	17.6 million	42.8 million	58.2 million
Percent distribution	100%	100%	100%
Aged (65 and over)	18.8	8.7	7.1
Blind and disabled	9.8	16.5	14.8
Adults in families with dependent children**	17.8	20.5	22.0
Children under age 21	44.5	46.1	47.8
Other***	9.0	8.6	8.4

*1972 is used instead of 1967, the first year of the program, because this is when the government began calculating the categories of people who receive benefits in contrast to those who are enrolled.
**Formerly persons who qualified for Aid to Families with Dependent Children (AFDC), which was abolished and replaced with the Temporary Assistance to Needy Families (TANF) program in 1997.
***Includes persons deemed medically needy by some states. This category fell to 1.7 percent of recipients by 1995, but has obviously increased since then.

Source: "Medicaid Recipients and Medical Vendor Payments, According to Basis of Eligibility, and Race and Ethnicity: United States, Selected Fiscal Years 1972–2000," *Health, United States, 2003: With Chartbook on Trends in the Health of Americans* (Hyattsville, MD: National Center for Health Statistics, 2003), table 137 (online at http://www.cdc.gov/nchs/data/hus/hus03.pdf); "Medicaid Beneficiaries and Payments, by Basis of Eligibility, and Race and Hispanic Origin: United States, Selected Fiscal Years 1999–2008," *Health, United States, 2010: With Special Feature on Death and Dying* (Hyattsville, MD: National Center for Health Statistics, 2011), table 143 (online at http://www.cdc.gov/nchs/data/hus/2010/143.pdf).

In interpreting quantitative material like this, it is always best to start by identifying the "biggest" facts. Look at who falls into the largest group of enrollees in table 6.1. It is adults with dependent children plus children under age twenty-one at a combined rate of 69.8 percent. Now look at table 6.2. Only 32 percent of payouts go for caring for poor adults and dependent children. The percent of enrollees who are aged or blind and disabled is 21.9 percent but 64.1 percent of expenditures go for their care. That is not

Table 6.2.   U.S. Medicaid Payments, 1972, 2000, and 2008

	1972	2000	2008
All payments	$6.3 billion	$168.3 billion	$294.2 billion
Percent distribution	100%	100%	100%
Aged (65 and over)	30.6	26.4	20.7
Blind and disabled	22.2	43.2	43.6
Adults in families with dependent children	15.3	10.6	12.7
Children under age 21	18.1	15.9	19.3
Other	13.9	3.9	3.9

Source: "Medicaid Recipients and Medical Vendor Payments, According to Basis of Eligibility, and Race and Ethnicity: United States, Selected Fiscal Years 1972–2000," *Health, United States, 2003* (Washington, DC: U.S. Department of Health and Human Services, Public Health Service, 2003), table 137; "Medicaid Beneficiaries and Payments, by Basis of Eligibility, and Race and Hispanic Origin: United States, Selected Fiscal Years 1999–2008," *Health, United States, 2010* (Washington, DC: U.S. Department of Health and Human Services, Public Health Service, 2010), table 143.

hard to understand, once you start thinking about it. A smaller proportion of children, even poor children who may not have the best diets and living conditions, are likely to require expensive care than the elderly and disabled who are more likely to be chronically ill. The fact that the number of elderly covered by Medicaid has been declining but the number of children covered by Medicaid has not changed deserves more attention.

If the number of elderly covered by Medicaid has declined, why does Medicaid spend so much on their care? The answer is that the money is largely spent on nursing home care. Remember that Medicare covers nursing home care for a limited period of time and only after hospitalization. What about people who need nursing care because they are chronically ill, frail, confused, need help medicating themselves, toileting, eating, and so forth? The determination that the person needs long-term nursing home care in such cases is made by the family, and a period of hospitalization may not be involved. How does nursing home care get paid for under these circumstances? Increasingly, people who are incapacitated enough to go into a nursing home, give up whatever money they have to their children, which makes them impoverished and eligible for Medicaid. The other alternative is to pay for it out of one's own pocket. Considering that, according to the Department of Health and Human Services, nursing home care averaged $219 per day or roughly $6,570 per month for a private room with no added services in 2009, while Medicaid coverage is free, you can understand why Medicaid has become a major alternative and is now providing coverage for an increasing number of people in nursing homes.[8]

The disabled category has been growing as well because increasing numbers of people are meeting the criteria for disability. Beyond being unable to work, applicants must prove that they are poor enough. Obviously, this means that they must have incomes below whatever the state has set up as the cutoff. That is considerably more complicated than it might first appear. What if a person receives a pension the person can live on, but runs up such high medical bills that he or she ends up being impoverished with very little money left to live on? This is called the "spend down" provision. A person may become eligible because so much of his or her money (e.g., social security check and/or pension) is going to pay for medical bills.

Consider the full implications of spending down. A person must cash in everything she owns before she can say she is truly impoverished. ("She" is appropriate here because there are more poor elderly women than men; because they outlive men, they bear the primary responsibility for supporting children, and they earn less, they have less of a savings cushion.) That, of course, means that the person can't own a house, a car that is worth more than whatever the state decides and so on. Finally, the person must prove that he or she is poor.

That is the "means testing" feature of the program. Means testing is used to determine whether a person is as poor as he or she claims to be. Accordingly, all financial records must be submitted to the state agency that carries out the review. The standard cutoff has long been $5,000 but is now $6,000 in some states, meaning that one must "cash in," typically giving to one's children everything that might put one's "wealth" over that line.

Critics of the Medicaid program have argued that this is a particularly objectionable feature of the program. They say that it is degrading and stigmatizing to have to prove that one is poor. Accordingly, many states no longer require proof that one has no wealth and even allow people to keep a car, if the income level is sufficiently low. There are also those who work with the Medicaid population who find no feelings of stigma on the part of Medicaid enrollees. Others object to the cost of checking to determine if people are eligible for government-covered health care services. Medicaid administrative costs are difficult to assess. However, it is not hard to see why administrative costs would be significant considering how much paperwork and clerical time is involved in attempting to verify eligibility. Administrators of clinics that provide health care to the poor say that about a third of the premiums, such organizations receive from government programs are wasted because they are used to cover the administrative costs of re-enrolling people.[9]

MEDICAID AND HEALTH CARE REFORM

Medicaid is scheduled to be expanded to all persons under age sixty-five with incomes under 133 percent of poverty as of 2014. This basically means that, adults with no dependent children and who are not pregnant, who have incomes under that poverty level, will be covered for the first time in many states. The law provided funding for states to extend Medicaid coverage to this population as of 2010. The 133 percent of the poverty rate creates a uniform eligibility standard across all states for the first time.

There has been a certain amount of resistance to this portion of the law because states are having difficulty meeting their budgets given the depth of the Great Recession the country is experiencing. In order to reduce resistance to compliance with the new law, the federal government is providing funds to cover 100 percent of the cost of health care services for those who are newly eligible from 2014 through 2016 and 95 percent in 2017, gradually dropping that rate over the following years to 90 percent by 2020. The rate the federal government will pay for the newly enrolled will stay at 90 percent over subsequent years. States that expanded eligibility to nonpregnant, childless adults prior to passage of the law will receive a phased-in increase in federal support.

The health care reform legislation makes it clear that undocumented illegal immigrants are not being covered by the expanded Medicaid law. In addition, the legislation provides 100 percent financing for primary care physician services in order to raise the level of reimbursement to the rate set by Medicare.

STATE CHILD HEALTH INSURANCE PROGRAM

The State Child Health Insurance Program (CHIP, referred to as SCHIP when it was legislated) or Title 21 of the Social Security Act is the third major public health program. It was passed in conjunction with the budget reform legislation of 1997. It was legislated in response to what we and everyone else who looks at health insurance and poverty data realized some time ago: that children, especially poor and near poor children, are at particularly high risk of being uninsured. CHIP provides federal funds to insure children under the age of nineteen whose family income is under 200 percent of the federal poverty level, which is much higher than the Medicaid cutoff in the majority of states. There is general support for providing health insurance for children; however, the challenge of enrolling children in families in which the adults are not poor enough to qualify for Medicaid has not been easy. States use three different models for establishing and administering CHIP: 1) a separate CHIP program, 2) Medicaid expansion, and 3) some combination of these. A 2004 estimate found that 32.1 million children were eligible, but only 44 percent of them were enrolled.[10] As of 2008, it was estimated by some that 7.3 million children were uninsured and of that number 65 percent were eligible for Medicaid or CHIP.[11] The number of enrolled children was reported to be 7.7 million as of 2010.

At the time the CHIP legislation was passed, Congress appropriated $40 billion over ten years that states could use to provide health care services for enrolled children with the provision that the states had to have administrative procedures in place and were already enrolling children. It took some states longer to do this than anticipated, which meant that allocated funds were not spent. That led to new controversies. A number of states that created CHIP programs more quickly applied for the unspent funds to cover childless adults. Some policy makers objected, saying that this was a distortion of the intent of the law. Congress dealt with the problem of unspent funds by passing a so-called "SCHIP Fix" in 2003 which allowed states to access some of remaining unspent funds. It appears that a great deal of attention was directed at analyzing the structure of the programs by state and distribution of these funds rather than measuring impact. That can be explained in part by the fact that there is general agreement that CHIP has been beneficial where it is operating effectively. The primary concern has been getting it to operate effectively.

QUESTIONS THAT REMAIN

The primary question that policy makers are confronting is how to cut the cost of these programs because the three public programs are now all being treated as entitlements and have been considered untouchable by politicians determined to cut government expenditures. However, the concern about public debt in Washington, D.C., if not the rest of the country, in the spring of 2011, has finally focused attention on the feasibility of cutting back on the costs of these programs. Let's consider some of the proposed solutions.

One of the options being explored is raising the age of eligibility to qualify for Medicare from sixty-five to sixty-seven in 2014. The following is based on a Kaiser Family Foundation Program on Medicare Policy report.[12]

Here are the facts. You can decide whether it would be a good move. Raising the age of eligibility by two years would generate an estimated $7.6 billion in net Medicare savings to the federal government. It would require a drop in coverage for about 5 million persons in this age bracket. However, it is projected that the savings would be offset by the $8.9 billion the government would have to spend for those who would then have to be covered by Medicaid; plus the $7.5 billion that the federal government would be providing in tax credits to those buying insurance through exchanges; and by the $7 billion reduction in Medicare premium receipts. The burden would shift $4.5 billion to employers who would still be the primary providers of insurance for their workers. Everyone buying insurance through exchanges, that would now include sixty-five- and sixty-six-year-olds, would pay 3 percent more for coverage because of increased risk of illness in the risk pool; Part B enrollees would also pay 3 percent more because younger Medicare recipients would be out of the risk pool; and states would have to spend $7 billion to provide Medicaid coverage for the new enrollees.

In short, Medicare expenditures would certainly drop. However, costs would not be eliminated; they would be shifted. That may be the really big lesson here. If your objective is to reduce government spending, to whom do you want to shift the costs? Who will support the shift, who will object, and how loudly will the interested parties on either side state their views?

Another alternative that is always there but tends not to attract much political support has moved to the forefront of the debate as of the spring of 2011. The proposition is to require prospective Medicare enrollees to purchase individual Medicare health insurance coverage in the market rather than have the government provide coverage. The argument as always is that the market will introduce much-needed efficiency—it will provide variety and choice so that enrollees can opt for plans that best suit their needs; and even more importantly, competition among insurers will reduce the cost of health insurance plans. What do you think? What is the evidence so far?

One set of facts should not go unnoticed in this part of the discussion. Do you recall that the reforms instituted by the ACA affecting private insurers limit profits and administrative costs, that is, the medical-loss ratio, to 15 percent? In this chapter we find that the administrative cost of running the Medicare program is 2 percent. So how is it more efficient to pay the difference, meaning 13 percent, to private insurance companies? Because market competition will certainly reduce the price of insurance plans? What is the evidence to support that assessment?

Less information is available on the costs of administering Medicaid and CHIP but we can be sure that the costs are higher than they are for Medicare because means-testing depends on a lot of record keeping and checking. That depends on high personnel costs in addition to health service costs.

There are a number of other more technical reforms of Medicare being discussed, such as reducing variation in payments by region of the country. And of course there are reforms that will affect delivery of care to all patients, not just Medicare patients.

· 7 ·

Opinions on the Health Care Reform Act

$\mathcal{S}$o what is your view of the Patient Protection and Affordable Care Act? Yes, we can all certainly agree that it is enormously complicated. Do you have any criteria in mind for making more specific judgments about it? Let's try to answer that question by looking at the law in light of the goals we want the health care system to strive for. It is also interesting to look at the results of polls asking other people about their reactions to the law. Since the law has given much of the responsibility to the market for overseeing the distribution of health insurance, let's end by reflecting on how well we expect that to work out.

WHAT DO WE WANT THE
HEALTH CARE REFORM LAW TO ACHIEVE?

The principal standard we seem to have for what we want the ACA to accomplish is how well it moves us closer to achieving the three goals our health care system sets forth—does it increase *access* to health care services, is it likely to improve the *quality* of care, and is it really designed to achieve *cost containment*? Is there anything more can we ask of it?

Access

As we saw in the last two chapters, the law does increase access by extending Medicaid to cover more people, by providing high-risk health insurance, and by subsidizing individuals and small businesses so that they can afford to buy private health insurance.

Quality

We have not devoted much attention to how the law proposes to improve the quality of care. Let's outline how it addresses this objective by identifying the new entities it has created to accomplish this.

- The Patient-Centered Outcomes Research Institute. This is a non-profit organization expected to identify research priorities and conduct research that compares the clinical effectiveness of medical treatments. It is designed to work under the auspices of a multi-stakeholder board. It is not authorized to set mandates or influence reimbursement.
- The National Prevention, Health Promotion, and Public Health Council created to coordinate federal prevention, wellness, and public health activities. The council will carry out this task in cooperation with the newly established community-based Collaborative Care Network Program, which is to give special attention to the needs of low-income persons.
- A more concrete step intended to benefit people's health is the determination that preventive services will be fully covered, that is, the co-payment for preventive services has been eliminated, under Medicare and Medicaid.
- Small employers interested in offering wellness programs will be eligible for grants to start such programs.
- Finally, the law requires chain restaurants and vending machine foods to have nutritional information for each item.

This review may not be comprehensive but it covers the most significant changes. So what do you think; does the law address quality to a sufficient extent?

Cost Containment

The third goal that our health care system aims to strive for, cost containment, is expected to be addressed via measures to be implemented under the auspices of the Medicare Program.

- The Independent Payment Advisory Board, which is mandated to submit legislative proposals designed to reduce the growth rate of Medicare spending if and when it exceeds a target growth rate.
- The Innovation Center within the Centers for Medicare & Medicaid Services (CMS), which is expected to test and expand payment structures while maintaining or improving quality of care.

- A Medicare pilot program to develop and evaluate paying a bundled payment for treatment by a physician, care in the hospital, and post-hospital care—coverage that begins three days prior to hospitalization and spans thirty days post-hospitalization.
- It prohibits payments to states for Medicaid services related to health-care-acquired conditions.
- It reduces payments for a variety of recipients, including Medicare Advantage plans, to hospitals for preventable readmissions and for hospital-acquired conditions.
- It reduces Disproportionate Share hospital payments to states with the lowest percentages of uninsured.
- It affects private insurance plans by imposing a single set of operating rules for eligibility verifications and claims status information in order to reduce expenses by simplifying administrative processes.

Before the law could go to Congress for a vote, the Congressional Budget Office (CBO) was required to calculate its impact on the budget. The CBO projected that health care reform would reduce the national deficit over the first ten years by $143 billion, and that this effect would continue over the following ten years but at a lower rate for a cumulative deficit reduction of about $1.5 trillion.[1]

Again, this is not a comprehensive review, but it does cover most of the changes. So, does the law address cost containment adequately?

No question about it, this part of the discussion adds a whole new layer of complexity to our understandings of what is in the law. And, as I have said before, we have no assurance that what the law intends will actually be implemented because so many parties are involved, some of whom have simply not made enough preparations to implement the law and others who are actively involved in resisting making the required changes. But now that you know more about how the law is supposed to work than most people in this country, what are your thoughts on how well the law addresses the goals we say we want our health system to strive for if not how well it will work? Perhaps seeing what other people think of it will help.

WHAT THE REST OF THE COUNTRY THINKS OF THE LAW

Let's stop for a moment and consider—is it possible that all the complaints that we have been hearing for such a long time about problems about our health system are just another example of media hype and that things really aren't so bad? Or are all those complaints coming from specific groups of people,

the elderly, for example, who really are particularly concerned about the effect of the law on Medicare and have the time to go to meetings with their
congressional representatives and tell them what they think? Maybe it is just
anti-government fringe groups? Or is it political activists at both ends of the
political spectrum who have been ranting and raving about these things? Yet,
as we all know, reports predicting either great improvements or great disasters
with the coming of health care reform would not be so common unless the
media watchers had established that such stories would attract large enough
audiences to convince sponsors to pay for advertising space.

The Political Split Prior to Passage of the ACA

Perhaps taking a closer look at how political party affiliation can explain the
extent of our dissatisfaction with prevailing arrangements will clarify things.
The general assumption is that party affiliation serves as a good indicator of
the way Congress will treat any piece of legislation. A 2008 review of surveys
focusing on political party preference indicates that there were significant
differences in attitude regarding the need for health care reform by political
party—46 percent of Democrats thought the system needed rebuilding but
only 28 percent of Republicans thought so.[2]

If the Democratic/Republican split suggests to you that we should be
grateful that so many people are declaring themselves to be independents, who
will be thoughtful and rational in their decisions rather than just following
the party line, political scientists warn us not to put much confidence in that
interpretation.[3] Political scientists who have examined the position taken by
independents tell us that the stance they take can be explained by the fact that
they are typically even less well-informed than those who identify with one
party or the other. Indeed, political scientists express a good deal of despon-
dency about how poorly informed the majority of Americans are about the
full range of issues they are asked about.

We might take some consolation if those who were less informed were
also less likely to vote. However, we have no reason to put our hopes on
that possibility. It turns out that it is the uninsured who are less likely to
vote. This fact had a significant impact on the outcome of the vote during
the last couple of elections when support for the health care reform being
promoted by the Democratic Party was on the agenda. The fact that so many
independents did vote and very few of the uninsured voted gave opponents
of health care reform, that is, the Republican Party candidates, particularly
Tea party candidates, an advantage in the mid-term election that took place
at the end of 2010.[4]

There is, however, more to the story on the split by political party affiliation. Consider the December 2009 survey results on what people thought of the health care reform proposal that was shaping up as reported by the CNN television network.[5]

42 percent in favor
39 percent opposed because they thought it was too liberal
13 percent opposed because they thought it was not liberal enough
6 percent other and no opinion

It looks like some of those who were opposed to the health care reform act thought it was not liberal enough. They had hoped that the reform plan would look more like a single-payer plan or a Medicare-for-all kind of plan for which the government would take full responsibility. We know that a number of congressmen said they would not vote for the 2010 reform bill precisely because it was not a single-payer plan and only reversed their votes at the last minute. (We will have a little more to say about the pros and cons of the single-payer plan shortly.)

In the end, the ACA did pass with a final vote in the House of Representatives of 291 to 212 without a single vote in favor by a Republican and with 34 negative Democratic votes. The Senate had to engage in some procedural maneuvering to get enough votes for passage. One of the stumbling blocks was resolved when coverage for abortions was dropped from the plan.

Public Opinion on ACA after It Was Passed

The Kaiser Family Foundation tracking poll, conducted less than two months after the law was passed in May of 2010, found that 41 percent of those surveyed registered positive views of the health care reform law, 44 percent held unfavorable views, and 14 percent were undecided or unsure.[6] Where people say they got their information on the law helps to clarify these results a bit—68 percent of respondents said they were getting their information from family and friends; 63 percent also mentioned cable, and 55 percent mentioned broadcast news programs. Of those who got their news from FOX News 78 percent were opposed to the law. Of those who watched CNN, 52 percent favored the law.

That the source of information is a major factor in whether Americans end up having a more favorable or less favorable stance toward the law is confirmed by the fact that a third of seniors responding to the poll were convinced that the government was creating "death panels" that would be making end-of-life care decisions for Medicare recipients. Those who were getting their information from FOX news were more likely to register opposition on this basis than those getting their information from CNN.

According to the Kaiser September 2010 poll, conducted six months after passage of ACA, 49 percent of Americans said they favored the law, 40 percent said they held an unfavorable view, but 53 percent of Americans also said they were confused about it.[7] Beyond that, a large majority said they were angry about the law. When asked what was making them angry, they reported that they were angry about the state of politics in Washington rather than the law itself. In fact, only about 11 percent of all respondents said that passage of the law would have a major effect on their vote during the mid-term elections that would be taking place two months later in November of 2010.

While the country may have been completely divided in how it perceived the law, a January 2011 poll found a high level of agreement on individual components of the law—approval for closing the Medicare doughnut hole (at 85 percent), approval for subsidies for low- and moderate-income Americans to buy health insurance (at 79 percent), approval for expanding the Medicaid program (at 67 percent).[8] The public was also pleased about the components that had already been put into effect by September of the year, including the fact that young adults could stay on their parents' plans until age twenty-six, that Medicare Part D enrollees whose pharmaceutical costs put them in the doughnut hole received checks in the mail for $250, and that the government had established an insurance plan for people who were defined as high-risk and uninsurable.

If the majority of Americans could find things they liked about the law, why so many continued to maintain negative view of the law as a whole requires additional careful analysis. The fact that the law is so complicated goes far in explaining how this might happen. To illustrate, when asked how they felt about the individual mandate, 76 percent of Americans said they were opposed, but when they were told that insurance companies are permitted to deny coverage to people who are sick and would continue to have this right unless the law required everyone to be insured and guaranteed that there would be insurance coverage for everyone, opposition dropped to 47 percent.

There is no question that Americans continued to be divided in their attitude toward the health care reform law well after it was enacted. It is also apparent that Americans were not becoming better informed with regard to the law and its implications. This is confirmed by the decision of the House of Representatives, which had a Republican majority after the mid-term elections, to schedule a vote to repeal the law. The vote was clearly a symbolic gesture since it was clear to members of the House of Representatives that the Senate, which retained its Democratic majority, would oppose the move and the president would reject it. In fact, the Senate never even put the measure to repeal the law on its agenda for discussion. However, the Kaiser Family Foundation poll taken in February of 2011 found that 22 percent of Americans thought the ACA had been repealed and 26 percent were not sure if it had been repealed or not.[9] In reporting the findings, Drew Altman, the president and CEO of the Kaiser Family Foundation, indicated that after all the polling the organization does, he was still very surprised and disappointed to find how ill-informed Americans are about the legislative process.

The Law as a Litmus Test of Divisions in this Country

Reflecting on the attitudes being expressed by Americans, where they say they get their information, and seeing how easily misinformation can spread, we would do well to take a step back and ask what is happening here. We saw evidence that the ACA was not really at the heart of this split in the American psyche when people said they were angry about that state of politics in Washington, D.C. So let's consider what else is going on to cause such a big political divide on first, passing and, second, on funding the health care reform act that we are seeing.

There is no question that the government's share of the health care bill will increase with passage of the ACA because more people will be eligible to enroll in Medicaid. The law is expected to increase the number of people covered by health insurance by 32 million according to the Congressional Budget Office (CBO) and 34 million according the Centers for Medicare & Medicaid (CMS) actuaries. The CMS calculated that it would save $828 billion, leaving a net overall cost of $251 billion, but did not consider revenue.[10] As we noted above, the CBO calculated that revenue and savings will more than offset costs over time. (I know these numbers are so large that they are incomprehensible so just remember that the CMS did *not* include revenue and the CBO *did* in projecting how the law would affect the national budget.)

Critics of the law are saying that the rise in health care spending means that the government will be responsible for over half of the nation's health care bill by 2012. And they say that is a sure sign of government takeover of the health care system. Is this really an effort to force out the private sector? Is that what is at the bottom of the split we see in Washington and in the rest of the country?

Implications of Health Care Reform from Different Disciplinary Perspectives

A number of very clear facts can be called upon to answer the questions I have just raised. Yes, the government will be paying for more of the bill, and, yes, the government will make every effort to implement the health care reform law in order to increase access, improve quality, and contain costs. Whether that can be interpreted to mean that it will be taking over our health care arrangements is a very different question. Let's consider some of the ways the government could take over the system and consider how likely that is to happen.

To begin with, there is no evidence in the law that the federal government intends to assume full control over the Medicaid program beyond setting a national standard for eligibility based on level of poverty. The fifty states will continue to be involved in managing their own Medicaid operations. They may choose to set up widely varying experimental adaptations in the effort to reduce costs, create programs to help people stay off Medicaid, and provide incentives to businesses to hire persons who would otherwise need various kinds of government support, including Medicaid coverage.

There is no evidence to indicate that the federal government is trying to abolish private insurance, only rein it in. The Medigap program provides an excellent illustration of how this can work without much opposition from any of the parties involved. The federal government was pleased to see private insurance companies create supplementary plans, but made sure that Medicare enrollees could understand what was in the plans they were purchasing when the private insurance companies began rolling them out.

Then there is the rising cost of Medicare. Let's use the proposal to increase the age of eligibility from sixty-five to sixty-seven discussed at the end of chapter six to see how observers coming at this issue from somewhat different perspectives might respond. Let's start with what economics has to offer since the issue has already been examined using one of the basic tools, namely, cost/benefit analysis. Utilizing this analytical tool we can assess current costs and projected costs against current and projected revenue and savings. That tells us that the savings to the Medicare Program that would accrue from increasing the age of eligibility would result in an impressive amount of money. But, as we saw, the savings look good at first, but stopping the analysis there would have been highly misleading. Shifting costs to other programs might or might not provide a good solution. In this case, the increased cost to other government and nongovernment programs would exceed any savings, which makes it a poor policy option for reducing Medicare costs from the perspective of economics. If politicians decide that raising the enrollment age does not provide a sufficiently effective solution—not that we can be sure that they will decide this—they will have to find other solutions. That will capture the attention of everyone likely to be affected, starting with the politicians themselves, whose chances of getting reelected will surely come into play.

The current commitment to rein in government spending and government oversight embraced by the most conservative branch of the Republican Party, the Tea Party, has resulted in a possible solution—a proposal designed to reduce Medicare spending by requiring future enrollees to purchase private health insurance policies. The idea is that Medicare enrollees would receive a voucher to procure their own insurance, but no assurance of health care coverage if they could not find a plan at a price covered by the voucher. The only other way that persons over the age of sixty-five could qualify for coverage would, of course, be by meeting Medicaid eligibility qualifications. It is not clear that proponents of the voucher alternative understand that this would raise government expenditures unless, of course, those who were eligible for Medicare would be prohibited from enrolling in Medicaid for some reason. Fear of this and other threatening similar possibilities is what is causing all those Medicare enrollees to confront politicians who are promoting this solution to see what the politicians have to say about it.

The question is whether commitment to a political agenda aimed at downsizing the role of government and favoring private sector solutions can withstand pressure from the sector of the population that would be affected and others who are opposed to making such a radical change in the Medicare program. Political scientists will surely be interested in exploring what various members of the public think of the Republican proposal. That has not happened at this writing.

Then there is the option of increasing the age of eligibility. That has received even less analytical attention so far. So we will have to suggest some of the questions that this perspective might produce. Sociologists might be interested in asking whether prospective retirees would delay retirement in order to maintain the insurance coverage they receive from their employers. That might lead to analysis of the impact that delayed retirement would have on young people just entering the labor force, whether fewer jobs would be available, and whether that, in turn, would have an impact on marriage and family. Such questions are obviously best considered from an interdisciplinary perspective. That would move us onto questions about the effects of reduced opportunities for occupational mobility and the impact on earnings of those who were not able to find a job. Such questions suggest bringing in researchers interested in the development of social capital and the impact that has on the country's productivity and national economy.

Doctors, especially those trained in public health who work on population health problems, not only health problems of individual patients, might be interested in studying the stress that increasing the age of eligibility has for the targeted age group and the implications that it is likely to have for their health indicators. That spills over into questions about the increased costs generated by the need to treat persons whose health is so affected. Of course, those in the age bracket just below the affected group would also be experiencing stress in anticipating how they will fare and how their health might be impacted with all the associated costs to which we have just alluded. Increased stress that affects some members of the family is certainly likely to affect other members of the family, and you can see how the implications could create expanding waves that researchers might be interested in documenting.

So now you see how it is that so many different disciplines have become involved in studying how the health care system operates. If you are interested in exploring these issues there are some very impressive interdisciplinary studies that I can recommend.[11]

WHICH APPROACH IS BETTER AT OVERSEEING THE SYSTEM?

Making adjustments to programs like increasing the age of eligibility for Medicare Program enrollees is complicated enough. Laying out the pros and cons of moving toward greater dependence on the market, by issuing vouchers on the one hand, to greater dependence on the government to oversee our health care arrangements on the other hand, is obviously even more complicated. Indeed, the intensity of the debate on whether the private sector or the public sector can do a better job of distributing health sector goods and services has been escalating in recent years.

The question is not whether everyone should have health insurance in this country. That is not the way the debate is presented. Even the most conservative members of society do not argue that it is okay for some people to be uninsured. What they register very strong feelings about is how people should obtain health insurance coverage. This is how the debate takes shape.

The essence of the argument is between those who favor the explanation espoused by economists who belong to the classical school of economics and economists who argue that the health care sector is a special case and does not fit the classical model. According to the classical school, the "invisible hand" of the market is a superior mechanism for distributing goods and services because it allows for flexibility in response to consumer demand; it adjusts quality and price in response to consumer preferences; and it offers only those products that consumers want. Having to shop for the products they want makes consumers more sensitive to the options that are available and more sensitive to costs. This has the effect of making consumers less likely to be wasteful in using goods and services, which keeps costs down for everyone. The invisible hand of the market serves a number of valuable functions. Sounds like a plan, doesn't it?

Let's consider the characteristics of an "ideal market":

- many sellers and many buyers resulting in steady and ongoing competition
- easy entry of new firms and exit of firms that fail
- excellent information for comparative shopping
- high responsiveness to pricing reflecting consumer preference
- constant innovation resulting in increasing value

Economists on the other side of this debate generally begin by referring to an article by Kenneth Arrow, the Nobel prize-winning economist, who outlined the reasons for treating health care as an exceptional case in 1963.[12] Let's begin with the fact that more than half of the population is still getting health insurance through their workplace; this means that most people are not actually shopping for insurance. They choose from the options presented by the employer, which the majority of employers have been reducing to an ever-smaller number of alternatives.

Economists who argue that the health market does not fit the ideal case say that health care is characterized by the following:

- the product is difficult to evaluate and, in some cases, may be so new that it still does not have a performance record.
- the seller (the physician) is the buyer's agent, controls information and moment of decision; moreover, buyers want it that way.
- shopping is costly and complex, not a sensible approach if other alternatives are available.
- medical services are not a product most people wish to purchase so the incentives are different.
- "utility theory" is difficult to satisfy because it requires that a person's priorities be clear, the benefits and risks be fully known, and, most important, that the buyer be able to keep all of this information in mind in order to make a rational choice.

Both proponents and critics agree that the free market operates on the principle of *caveat emptor*, which translates into "buyer beware." However, they interpret the advantages and disadvantages involved differently. Proponents say that it makes buyers more sensitive to cost and prevents *moral hazard*. Moral hazard is a term that economists use to capture the idea that many of us cannot resist the temptation to use products and services that are free even if we don't need them. It is true that some people will take advantage of treatments that they do not really need; on the other hand, how many of us have time to indulge or interest in indulging in that kind of thing?

The big exception to this observation can be found in how we respond to the invitation to consume pharmaceuticals. Many of us can't wait to use the drugs that promise to help us breathe better, lift our mood, and give us a wonderful sleep, not to mention what drugs can do for our sex lives. So moral hazard may well apply when it comes to pharmaceuticals but not so much when it comes to other medical goods and services. A great deal can be said about the pharmaceutical industry that we do not have the space to get into. I can recommend some excellent books on the topic.[13]

Let's go back to the role that invisible hand plays. Is it really an efficient and equitable mechanism for distributing goods and services that eliminates government interference and more importantly rationing by the government? According to Rashi Fein, a medical economist who has been working in this field for quite some time, the invisible hand does not eliminate rationing at all. It merely changes who is doing the rationing.[14] The invisible hand rations by allowing private sector organizations to make health care services too expensive for some portion of the population. Eliminating the people who cannot afford to pay for health care from the market makes services more accessible to those who are in a position to pay for what they want.

That brings me back to a question that came up in the first chapter to which I said I would return later, namely, why do people from other countries come here for health care? Doesn't that prove that it is the best health system in the world? My answer is that they do so to get around the "queue," that is, the waiting line. In most countries, the doctors decide whose case is most urgent and should be dealt with first. In this country, there are always ways to get ahead of the line. Individuals, including foreigners, can and do get the services they want, if they are willing to pay for that privilege. What do you think? What are the pros and cons of making excellent and expedient health care services available to foreigners as well as fellow Americans who are in a better position to pay for those services? Would you say that this might have the effect of pushing some Americans to the end of the line or out of the line entirely?

Getting back to the *caveat emptor* principle, those who are opposed to reliance on competition in the health sector say that this is the wrong principle on which to base health care arrangements. Opponents have also argued that competition does not increase efficiency and reduce costs; rather, it produces inefficiencies by creating instability and waste. This happens when established and familiar organizations are sold or merge with other organizations. That brings new faces and new rules and this reduces efficiency as the new organizations become established, adopt new procedures, replace staff, and so on. Remember what was happening before the HMO market settled down?

A competitive environment does encourage beneficial innovation. Yet, it also promotes negative innovation, that is, the development of fraudulent products and services. It encourages testing the limits of utility and legality, which is, of course, why the *caveat emptor* warning exists. The prevention of shady practices and outright fraud requires a great deal of costly monitoring. That explains, in part, why the administrative costs are so much higher under competitive arrangements than they are under noncompetitive arrangements like the arrangements that exist in so many advanced societies—that, plus the amount of money that is going to the CEO, other executives, and shareholders. After all, the for-profit designation means that there has to be a margin of profit—the bigger the better.

THE SINGLE-PAYER ALTERNATIVE

At the opposite end of the spectrum are those who not only want to reduce the extent to which our health care system depends on competition but they also want a system in which competition has no part. These are the folks who support the single-payer plan. Given that the health care reform law explicitly rejected this option, let's take a brief look at what that kind of plan might look like. A single-payer proposal was thoroughly outlined by the Physicians' Working Group for Single-Payer National Health Insurance in a 2003 article in the *Journal of the American Medical Association*.[15] It is based on four principles:

- insurance coverage should not be tied to employment.
- the right to choose a physician is fundamental.
- corporate profit has no place in caregiving.
- medical decisions should be determined by patients and doctors, not corporations or government bureaucrats.

The authors say that "The United States alone treats health care as a commodity distributed according to the ability to pay, rather than as a social service to be distributed according to medical need."[16] They argue that the advantages of providing universal access are obvious. Not only would people be healthier and more productive if they were assured that they could get health care when they needed it, they would not run up high costs resulting from delayed care. The authors note that half of bankruptcies in this country are attributable to medical debt. They say that data on bankruptcies is difficult to find because debt may be charged to credit cards, may be financed through second mortgages, may go to collection agencies, and so on. However, when those going through bankruptcy are surveyed, 78 percent report medical debt.[17]

The authors of the single-payer proposal maintain that eliminating private insurance would result in an immediate drop in health care expenditures because administrative costs would decline sharply. They point out that private health insurance consumes 12 percent of premiums on average, whereas Medicare consumes about 3 percent. (The most recent figure is a 2 percent administrative cost.) They also say that the percent of the premium for administration of individual health insurance plans is far greater than is generally reported, up to 45 percent of the premium in some instances.

By the way, do you recall the *New York Times* poll we discussed in chapter two that found that 72 percent of Americans would like to see a "Medicare for all" type of plan instituted?[18] That is exactly what a single-payer plan is. It is interesting to see this much support for a single-payer plan on the one hand and so much opposition to government control over health insurance on the other hand. Hard to explain, but, I do think the issue deserves a closer look.

Accuracy of Estimates of Health Care Costs

We know that Americans pay much more for health care than people in other countries. But two of the authors of the single-payer plan article argue elsewhere that the government's health care cost burden is being underestimated. They say that the only costs being considered are direct government expenditures on Medicare, Medicaid, Veterans Administration, public health, and hospital subsidies. They contend that the tax subsidies that government extends to employers for offering insurance and expenditures on public employee health insurance costs should be included. This more accurate calculation, they say, raises the government share of health care costs to 59.8 percent rather than the 45.3 percent the government reports.[19] Thus, they say the government's contribution is actually a matter of "public funding" plus "tax financing." In short, they advocate eliminating this tax loss and using the additional funds this would produce to fund a national health care plan. Another way of looking at it is that we are already spending nearly as much as countries that have national health programs.

Calculating how much we are spending compared to how much we are losing by tolerating such a high level of uninsurance, the Institute of Medicine reports that the economic losses stemming from lack of health insurance in 2004 amounted to $65 to $130 billion a year due to higher disease and death rates among the uninsured.[20] The IOM maintained that there will be no increased cost resulting from extending health insurance to everyone since the rate of economic loss that is the result of people not working to their full capacity is higher than the estimated cost of providing insurance for all Americans.

Finally, there is the question of whether we think that having a two-tier or multiple tier system of health care is likely to result in continuing efforts to extend the health insurance coverage to those who will be able to purchase only the most basic plans. In other words, it would not be surprising to find people deciding that better health insurance will lead to better health care and that this is directly correlated to the variation in health status and life expectancy. Given that interpretation, what are the chances that more energy will be devoted to changing the system in order to achieve better insurance for that portion of the population covered by plans that are less generous?

When Costs Started to Rise

What I would like to add to this commentary is that it would be good to get a better sense of when our health care costs started to increase so much, indeed, increase at a much greater pace than they were increasing in other countries. We will discuss the health care systems in other countries in the next chapter. For now, I want to focus on what was happening in this country when the rate of increase in U.S. health care costs started to diverge from the rate of increase other countries were experiencing. That happened around 1980. We can see a number of other trends taking off around this time as well. This is when our sense of trust in each other and in our social institutions started to decline at a faster rate than it had been declining since we began collecting that information in 1969. Remember that, as we discussed in chapter two, according to some observers the lack of trust in social institutions and government goes a long way in explaining why the country is so divided in its assessment of health care reform. Wilkinson and Pickett provide us with charts documenting this trend.[21] The charts also show that this is also when economic inequality started to increase.[22]

What was happening in this country around 1980 that coincides with trends that started to ascend around that time? One answer is that this is when the message that the private sector, more specifically the for-profit sector, could get the job done more efficiently than government or nonprofit organizations took off in a big way. The underlying rationale was that monetary incentives would motivate people to do their best work, which those on Wall Street quickly translated into the memorable slogan: "Greed is Good."

How is this related to the rise in health care costs? You can say that Americans suddenly became more interested in seeking more health care around this time and that this explains why costs increased. However, that explanation works only if you follow that up by arguing that people in other economically advanced societies were not nearly as interested in seeking health care services, which is certainly not true. The point I want to emphasize is that the pace of the rise in health care costs in this country over the last three decades has been much greater than it has been in other countries. We are now paying twice as much for our health care than people in the top fifteen advanced countries.[23] And remember that those countries have been providing health care coverage for all their citizens while we have been leaving at least 18 percent of our fellow Americans uninsured.

In my view you really can't miss seeing a pattern—we turned to the for-profit sector approach starting around 1980 because the country bought into the promise on the part of those who were telling us that for-profit organizations were capable of delivering health insurance and other health care goods and services more efficiently and effectively. The message just got louder as evidence continued to mount that costs were increasing at an unprecedented rate in this country. Costs did increase in other countries, but they did so at a much slower rate. Virtually all economically advanced countries managed to stabilize the rate of increase at around this time. We did not. And, as we will see in the following chapter, it is not that all those countries rejected private sector participation; it is just that they have not been as ready to buy into the for-profit mantra to the same extent.

It is hard to understand why Americans are willing to believe projections presented by believers in for-profit solutions promising that costs will decline in the future if we just give market competition enough time. That is the story we have been hearing for the last three decades and all the while costs have continued to rise, and at a faster pace than in all those other countries that have not chosen to use the for-profit approach.

If this suggests to you that I think that the whole issue of health care reform is far from settled, you are reading that right. And, since we cannot predict how well implementation of health care reform will go, perhaps we should now turn our attention to how other countries handle health care rather than dwelling on how disillusioning it has been to consider how Americans are dealing with health care and what that says about the country's mind-set in general.

· 8 ·

The Health Care Systems
in Other Countries

$\mathcal{I}$n the first chapter, I noted that Americans keep saying that ours is the best health care system in the world in spite of the fact that we don't live as long, we have a higher infant mortality, and we pay a great deal more for our health care than people do in many other countries. So who does have the best health system in the world and how do we determine that?

THE UNITED STATES COMPARED TO OTHER COUNTRIES

The expense involved in carrying out international surveys prevents pollsters from conducting them on a regular basis, but those that have been carried out are especially informative. The results of a comparative international study, reported in 1990, are particularly striking. A random sample of people in ten advanced, industrialized countries were asked to evaluate their health care arrangements (including Canada, the Netherlands, France, West Germany, Australia, Sweden, Japan, England/Wales, Italy, and the United States).[1] Compared to people in all those other highly industrialized countries, Americans were at the low end of the spectrum on satisfaction at that time. While the correlation is not perfect, it seems that the more a country spent on health care, the more satisfied the people were with their health care arrangements. The United States was the major exception. To reiterate, we were spending the most on health care and we were the least satisfied—and of course we were not living as long.

The most recent international comparative study at this writing was conducted in 2007. While the survey explored a wide range of issues, I would like to draw your attention to the satisfaction/dissatisfaction question once again.

Table 8.1.   Health System Views and Cost Among Adults in Seven Countries*

	Dissatisfaction (percent)	GDP (percent)	Life expectancy M	Life expectancy F
Australia	18	8.7	78.5	83.3
Canada	12	10.0	78.0	82.7
Germany	27	10.6	76.7	82.0
Netherlands	9	9.5 (2004)	77.2	81.6
New Zealand	17	8.0 (2003)	77.9	81.9
United Kingdom	15	8.4	77.2	81.5
United States	34	15.3	74.9	79.9

* All data is from 2006, except where noted.

Sources: On dissatisfaction: Cathy Schoen et al., "Toward Higher-Performance Health Systems: Adults' Health Care Experiences in Seven Countries, 2007," *Health Affairs* 26 web exclusive (2007), w717–34. On the GDP: "Total Health Expenditures as a Percentage of Gross Domestic Product, and Per Capita Health Expenditures in Dollars, By Selected Countries: Selected Years 1960–2006," *Health, United States, 2009: With Special Feature on Medical Technology* (Hyattsville, MD: National Center for Health Statistics, 2010), table 122 (online at http://www.cdc.gov/nchs/data/hus/hus09.pdf). On life expectancy: "Life Expectancy at Birth and at 65 Years of Age, by Sex: Selected Countries and Territories, Selected Years 1980–2005," *Health, United States, 2009: With Special Feature on Medical Technology* (Hyattsville, MD: National Center for Health Statistics, 2010), table 23 (online at http://www.cdc.gov/nchs/data/hus/hus09.pdf).

Respondents were given three options in reporting their level of dissatisfaction: 1) only minor changes needed; the system works well, 2) fundamental changes needed, and 3) rebuild completely. Table 8.1 reports the percentage of those who chose the third option—rebuild completely—as well as GDP and life expectancy statistics.

As you can see, Americans are again more dissatisfied, paying more, and not living as long as people in other countries. Let's consider what indicator we would like to use to determine what is, in fact, the best health care system in the world. Is it satisfaction or do you think we might come up with a better indicator?

Perhaps we should use life expectancy as the single most important indicator. Then, we would conclude that Japan has the best health care system. However, Americans are quick to say that the Japanese have a very different lifestyle than we do, which probably accounts for their longevity, but that we are not ready to adopt their values and lifestyle. In other words, there is little interest in promoting the Japanese model in this country. If we use infant mortality as the indicator, we find that Iceland and Singapore have an even lower rate than Japan (at 1.8 infant deaths in Iceland, 2.3 in Singapore, and 2.6 in Japan). Again, these countries are not considered to be appropriate models.

If we use health expenditures, we find that the cost of care per person in this country in 2008 was $7,538, according to the Organization for Economic Co-operation and Development (OECD). That is nearly double the average per person expenditure in the fifteen most highly developed countries, which averaged $3,923.

As we noted in the first chapter, one of the things that Americans seem to be particularly proud of when they talk about how good the health care system is in this country is our high-tech machines, particularly our CT (computed tomography) scanners and our MRI (magnetic resonance imaging) units. According to the OECD data collected in 2006 on thirty-three countries, we did have more CT scanners than many European countries: 34 per million people in the population compared to the UK, which had 7.6. On the other hand, Australia reported having 56 per million people and Japan had 97.3 per million (in 2008).

Americans do not realize that CT scanners were invented in England. Most Americans would be far more surprised to hear that when a group of English businessmen decided to chip in and buy more CT scanners and present them to the National Health Service (NHS) some years ago, the NHS said, "No thank you; we don't need more." The NHS said the scanners would just drive up costs without producing better health.

Where does that leave us with regard to the value we place on our high-tech capacity? The Japanese as well as most Europeans have longer life expectancies than we do, although they have vastly different numbers of high-tech machines—doesn't that make it hard to argue that our system is better because we have superior technology? Maybe a composite measure that includes cost, access, and quality, which we say are the goals of our system, plus patient satisfaction, would provide a better indicator. Using this composite measure, the World Health Organization has determined that France has the best health care system.

When policy makers in this country discuss the changes that we need to make to improve our health care system, they typically refer to a small number of European countries and Canada to make comparisons, but generally not France. Those who have reason to be interested in health care reform have been eager to point out what is wrong with health care arrangements in virtually all other countries and to argue that we would be making a big mistake if we imported any of those arrangements. However, they have said that arrangements developed by a few countries might have some lessons to offer. Some observers enthusiastically promoted the Swiss health care system during the years following the collapse of the Clinton proposal. However, that did not last, when it became clear that the Swiss system was the third most expensive system across economically advanced countries and that their out-of-pocket costs were the highest across developed countries.

Once preparations for the 2008 presidential elections started to take shape and it became clear that the Democrats were once again placing health care reform at the top of their political agenda, talk went back to what is wrong with the health care arrangements in the countries that we have spent so much time trashing—Canada and the UK. The worst charge that critics can launch at Canada and the UK is that their health care systems are socialistic. As we all know that is meant to invoke images of failure, grinding bureaucracy, and incompetence. Let's examine those systems a little more closely plus a few others that attracted the attention of policy experts and politicians alike. Since it is the Canadian system that consistently inspires more heated debate in this country than the systems in other countries, we'll look at their arrangements first.

Canada

In 2008, Canadians paid $4,079 per person for their health care services. The men were living to 78 and the women living to 82.7. By comparison, the United States was spending $7,538 per person; men were living to 74.9 and women to 79.5. You have to admit, they must be doing something right.

Canada has ten provinces, which are like our states but more independent of the federal government than American states, and three territories (the Yukon Territory, the Northwest Territories, and Nunavut). The foundation for the present health care system was laid in 1867 when the federal government gave the provinces responsibility for health care. However, the Canadian system really took shape during the 1940s. The province of Saskatchewan was the first to enact a provincial hospital insurance plan in 1947. In 1957, the federal government passed legislation establishing a national program to which the provinces would have to sign on and agreed to pay for half of the costs. By 1961, all the provinces had adopted the plan. The financial windfall of federal support caused Saskatchewan to propose a new program to cover medical care costs (i.e., doctors' fees). The doctors were not happy about the hospital plan; however, they were vehemently opposed to the medical portion of the plan. They said that this was the beginning of socialized medicine, which would cause quality to decline, costs to go up because of mismanagement, and treatments to be determined by bureaucrats. The citizens of the province thought otherwise. Saskatchewan introduced medical insurance in 1961. The other provinces followed. And, by 1971, Canada had a National Health Insurance Program it called Medicare.

The Canadian Medicare plan has a number of distinguishing features. It is generally referred to as a "single-payer" plan. The single payer is, of course, the government. Coverage must be comprehensive as specified by federal law, but additional services, such as dental benefits, home care, and drugs, are offered at the discretion of the province. The vast majority of hospitals are privately owned and operated by nonprofit organizations. Most doctors are paid on a fee-for-service basis, although an increasing number are opting to be paid on a salary basis. Patients are free to choose any primary care doctor they want. Canadians are issued a Medicare card, which is like a credit card. Patients are not billed, because the doctor's charges are reimbursed directly by the government.

We have a lot in common with Canadians. We share a very lengthy border. We speak the same language. We have similar historical roots. People in other countries can't tell us apart from the Canadians. So if we are so much like them and their health care arrangements are superior to ours in many ways—they spend less than we do, everyone is fully covered, they live a little longer than we do, and they seem to be quite satisfied—why don't we just copy it and be done with it? The answer is that no matter how alike we seem to be on the outside, the Canadian plan reflects their values, which are not our values. Even if some people in this country would like for the United States to embrace their values, that is not the way it works. Consider some of the objections heard in this country.

In the Canadian system everyone is covered by the same plan, which means you cannot buy more, faster, or better care. Americans refuse to accept that kind of arrangement. It is true that some Canadians have argued against it as well, but the vast majority of Canadians like things just the way they are. The position of the majority is that, when everyone is in the same boat, that boat is likely to be much better cared for. In other words, it is always easier to deny funding to "them," but when it is "us" whose care is at stake, "we" tend to exhibit more concern and readiness to treat the topic of the need for increased funding more seriously. Selling private health insurance for anything the government covers was made illegal with the passage of Medicare. Accordingly, you can buy more of anything the government does not cover—better wheelchairs, eyeglasses, even more amenities in your hospital room. That feature came into question in 2005 when the Canadian Supreme Court determined that Quebec's law prohibiting the sale of insurance for services covered by Medicare was illegal. How that is working out is still not entirely clear.

Canadians debate what they call "privatization" of services, which is what we call for-profit health care services governed by market forces, that is, competition. The same arguments prevail, namely, that for-profit sector organizations are superior, less expensive, and more attentive to consumer preferences. Access to faster service for a fee has received greater attention in recent years because of growing dissatisfaction with the length of waiting times. Proponents of privatization say that for-profit facilities and services would reduce waiting times for everyone by cutting down the length of the lines in the public system. Opponents argue that anything that is not accessible to the entire population violates the spirit of the law that created the Canadian Medicare system. Some evidence indicates a slight shift in readiness, especially among younger Canadians, to consider user fees for the most rapidly expanding sectors, especially newer forms of technology and home care.[2] The growing number of free-standing for-profit CT and MRI clinics which provide imaging services that people must pay for out of their own pockets directly rather than through additional insurance indicates that privatization is, in fact, moving ahead.

The length of waiting time for CT and MRI scans is related to another significant feature of the Canadian system, which is the "cap" on funding. Each year the provincial government sets a health care budget. Hospitals receive a fixed amount of money that covers basic operating expenses plus inflation, but they must negotiate any major expenses separately. The province's economic health determines how generous the province is in agreeing to additional hospital expenditures for technology and other kinds of upgrades.

Doctors do not have to negotiate over fees from year to year. Their fees are reimbursed in full for all the charges they submit. Why doesn't this result in unlimited charges? One reason is that doctors, particularly specialists, have increasingly been opting to be reimbursed on a non-fee-for-service basis. They sign a fixed annual contract with the hospital where they do most of their work. Those who rely on fee-for-service reimbursement accept lower levels of reimbursement after reaching specified income levels in some but not all provinces. As of 2004, doctors in Ontario, which is the richest province, agreed to accept 75 percent of the scheduled fee after they reach $465,000. Doctors' fee schedules are determined through negotiation between each respective provincial government and provincial medical society. The provincial government does not run out of funds for the year because it has budgeted what it will be spending based on the record of expenditures over the previous year and the revenue it expects to collect.

American doctors have traditionally considered Canadian reimbursement arrangements to be an unacceptable intrusion on the part of the government. Canadian doctors see it as preferable to the constant "micromanagement" that American doctors have to endure from insurance companies. American doctors have had to get preapproval from patients' insurance companies for many procedures in order to be sure the insurance plan covers the procedure and that they will be paid for performing it. Because there are so many plans with so many variations in coverage, which may change at any time, doctors' organizations in this country have periodically issued statements indicating support for the single-payer approach.

Another reason Canadian doctors are willing to accept a cap on income or a set salary has to do with two notable differences in expenses doctors face in the United States versus Canada. U.S. doctors are much more likely to enter into practice with a large educational debt. Canadian medical schools are heavily subsidized by the government, meaning that medical school tuition runs anywhere from $3,000 to $15,000 or so per year, depending on the province, compared to $60,000 to $125,000 per year in the United States. Also, malpractice insurance has been much lower. In part, this is because contingency fees are considered unethical or illegal in Canada. (Remember the contingency fee that goes to lawyers in this country is generally a third or quarter of the settlement, depending on whether the case is settled in or out of court, and no fee if they lose the case.)

Canadians find themselves periodically arguing about the performance of their health care system because the provinces have, from time to time, had to decide whether they wanted to come up with additional funding or cut services. The federal contribution to health care costs, which was 50 percent originally, was initially cut during the 1980s finally dropping down to 25 percent by the early 1990s. As you might imagine, talking about how to compensate for lost funds opened up public debate with the question of where the money should come from. This led to highly charged questions about what should be cut to lower costs and whether to allow more health care services to be offered for an additional charge. The fact that Canada was faced with an economic recession during the early 1990s led to the fear that the health care system was threatened. The economy improved during the last years of the twentieth century. In 1999, the federal government announced a fiscal surplus, which everyone agreed should go to the provinces to cover Medicare.[3]

As concern about funding declined during the first decade of the twenty-first century so has the volume of debate about how to best save the health care system. Polls have long found Canadians expressing strong support for maintaining the status quo on the essence of the single-payer arrangement, meaning they overwhelmingly reject two-tier care and user fees for core services.

To sum up, the most important differences between the Canadian system and ours is that theirs is a single-payer, capped system, while ours depends on market forces and competition to control costs; theirs provides health care coverage for everyone, ours has not; and theirs costs less than ours. These points speak to costs and access, but what about quality? Their life expectancy and infant mortality rates are better than ours. This, of course, just scratches the surface of things that people can argue about in discussing the differences between their system and our system.

At this point, let's turn to England to see how their health care system compares to ours.

England

In 2008, England was spending $3,129 per person on health care services. The men were living to 77.2 and the women to 81.5.

England, Scotland, Wales, and Northern Ireland together make up the United Kingdom or UK. Because the health care systems are not identical throughout the UK, the following discussion focuses on England, where health insurance for workers came into existence about 1911. Health care for the rest of the family was the family's responsibility. The logic is clear. Remember, England was the place the industrial revolution began. The industrialists were interested in making sure that their workers were healthy. Their main concern was workforce stability, not anyone's health per se, and certainly not the health of persons who were not their employees.

The emergence of hospitals in England has a longer history. This history serves as a particularly graphic illustration of how social values influence the development of social institutions.[4] Hospitals were established several centuries ago (some as early as the sixteenth and seventeenth centuries) with the express purpose of serving three separate segments of the population. The aristocracy went to sanatoriums, which were located in the countryside where the patients could benefit from clean air and the special comforts the rich expected. The working poor (i.e., all workers, in contrast to the aristocracy who do not work even now) went to voluntary hospitals often operated by religious orders. That left the "undeserving poor" (i.e., those who were too sick, too old, or too disabled to work). Because the aristocracy would not mix with the working poor and neither would mix with the undeserving poor, each segment had to have its own hospital. All that changed with World War II.

During the war, the government mapped out all the hospitals and counted all the hospital beds in the country and mandated that 10 percent of the beds in each hospital be set aside for military use. The hospitals were paid a *per diem* (daily) rate whether the bed was in use or not. Everyone in the country was making sacrifices. This was the hospitals' contribution to the war effort. While the country came out of the war victorious, it sustained heavy damage and was broke. The government proposed taking over responsibility for the entire health care system as a reward to the public for making enormous sacrifices during the wartime period. In other words, from that time on, the government took over ownership of the whole health care system. Not everyone was entirely happy about this plan. Doctors were especially loud in their objections. They said the government's plan was socialized medicine and would bring with it the downfall of professional medical practice. Looking at it objectively, it was, for better or worse, a major step toward socialized medicine. Doctors objected to being salaried instead of being paid as professionals under the traditional fee-for-service arrangement. On the other hand, one has to be practical in these matters. Having the government provide a guaranteed income was not easy to dismiss given the post-war state of affairs.

The solution was interesting. The general practitioners agreed to be paid under a *capitation* arrangement. They acceded to having X number of patients (around 2,000, more or less, depending on whether the practice was in an urban or rural area) sign up with them for care and get paid "by the head" (i.e., capitation) whether those patients came to see them or not. This meant that the doctors were guaranteed a steady income. The patients were guaranteed the services of a doctor. Patients had the opportunity to change doctors once a year by signing up with a new doctor of their choice. The specialists made a different bargain. They agreed to be salaried and work for a particular hospital in return for having access to 10 percent of the beds in that hospital for their private patients, whom they could bill separately. Everyone else working in the hospital had always been salaried, so that did not change.

In short, England has had a National Health Service, the NHS (not a national health insurance system), since 1948, with everyone in the country having full access to health care services. In assuming responsibility for the hospitals as of 1948, the government took over ownership of all the hospitals and clinics. It pays everyone who works for the NHS. How happy is everyone involved? How can you tell? When asked, the British have said that the health care system is second only to the monarchy in popularity.[5] This should not be taken to mean that they don't complain about the system. A more concrete way of assessing satisfaction is to count how many people opt out of the system. In the case of doctors, how many choose to leave to practice elsewhere? The critics of the NHS say that doctors are leaving in droves. In actuality, it is difficult to know how many leave and for what reasons. There is no count of how many leave and return after some period of postgraduate education or research outside the country (not always to the United States). To the extent that evidence exists, very few doctors are leaving.

In the case of patients, the measure is how many choose to buy private insurance and go to private doctors and hospitals. Until the 1980s, only about 5 percent of the population chose to buy private insurance. By the early 1990s, about 15 percent had done so. That figure has not changed much since then. How should we interpret this? It certainly indicates some growth in dissatisfaction, but not wholesale growth, right? Another catch here is worth noting.

When people buy private insurance, they buy it on top of having access to care through the National Health Service. What advantage are people seeking in buying private insurance if they have access to free care? Better doctors, better technology, more care? Not exactly. The answer is—getting around the "queue," in other words, waiting in line. In order to keep costs down, the NHS prevented people from getting health care services "on demand" (i.e., whenever they feel like it) for problems that are not life-threatening. In other words, people must wait while more urgent cases are treated. Those who feel that the wait is too long, and can afford to do so, buy private insurance. One of the most often cited reasons for doing this has been hip replacement surgery. It is painful, but not life-threatening.

Now for the essence of the "catch" I mentioned earlier. Private hospitals, where patients with private insurance go, do routine surgeries, like hip replacements. (I know, not routine to the person having the surgery, but routine in terms of how often it is done, and how much risk is involved.) If something does go seriously wrong, the patient is picked up by ambulance and taken to a major NHS hospital, which is equipped to deal with high-risk and complicated problems. So everyone is happy, right? Well, not entirely.

The reason that people have been buying private insurance is that the government kept the budget for the NHS low—much too low, in the opinion of some. (England has been spending a little less than half of what we spent for the last two decades of the twentieth century as reflected in percentage of GDP.) Couldn't the British alter this? After all, it is their social institution; they created it, they can change it, right? That is true. But remember this is the NHS, not an insurance plan. Its budget is in the hands of the ruling political party in office, which is elected by the public. In theory, the public should be able to convince the government to respond to its demands and allocate more funds for this purpose. The public did demand increased funding during the 1980s, and on one or two occasions the government did respond, but only after an enormous amount of public protest. The NHS did not receive a major infusion of funds until 1998. That happened because the British chose to elect a new prime minister in 1997, Tony Blair, who promised to put more liberal policies in place, including allocating more funding for the health care system. Since people must weigh their dissatisfaction with the way one social institution is being treated by the government against how they think other social institutions are faring, they may not be so eager to oust the current party until they are unhappy enough about all of it. They are more apt to try to convince the government via appeals and protests first. In 1997, British citizens did determine that electing a more liberal political party to office would improve the health care system as well as other social arrangements and institutions.

The newly elected prime minister was true to his word.[6] His objective was to raise the NHS budget from the 6.8 percent of GDP spent in 1997 to 9.4 percent by 2007–2008. He made clear that he would reverse the changes introduced during the two previous Conservative Party administrations, who had been impressed with U.S. efforts to introduce competition in order to increase efficiency. The mechanism the Conservative administrations had developed to promote greater efficiency was "fund holding." This gave general practitioners the option of managing their own funds and spending the monies they saved in running the practice on anything the practice group wanted to purchase. (They could not keep the surplus as a bonus.) Policy makers were somewhat surprised to find that the groups used the funds to ensure that social services were more closely aligned with medical services. The American way would have been to spend it on more technology and more expensive furnishings for their offices to attract more patients—right? It just goes to show how cultural values shape social institutions and why they vary from one country to another.

The newly elected prime minister stated that he was abolishing fund holding, in order to promote greater cooperation rather than competition. The change turned out to be largely semantic. What changed was what physician practice groups were called—from Fund Holders to Primary Care Trusts. Additionally, participation became compulsory. A number of other more sweeping changes followed. New diagnostic and treatment centers were opened to reduce waiting times. A National Institute for Clinical Excellence was established and mandated to issue binding recommendations on the delivery of medical services funded by the NHS. Doctors were now required to go through relicensure every five years. The latter two changes occurred in reaction to the death of a number of children, the result of cardiac surgeons doing operations outside of their competence, which outraged the British public. The performance of each Primary Care Trust was to be rated on a star basis—zero to three—and rewarded with increased autonomy or punished through increased managerial oversight, depending on the number of stars earned. The intent was to encourage peer review and adherence to evidence-based clinical guidelines. Three-star trusts, designated "foundation trusts," were given far greater independence, allowing them to raise capital on their own rather than being totally dependent on the national treasury. All trusts were expected to move in this direction eventually.

As of April 2004, general practitioners were permitted to choose among a number of contractual incentive arrangements for the first time, including capitation with incentives for reaching particular service targets, for example, a higher vaccination rate. This was part of an effort to reach ten specific targets for quality improvement, such as reducing cancer deaths by 20 percent. Contracts with specialists, called "consultants" in England, have changed only to the extent that NHS patients were now permitted, for the first time, to schedule their own appointments with specialists online.

In spite of all the changes introduced and money invested in the NHS by the Blair government during the late 1990s, 69 percent of the British public said that the government was not improving things enough and physicians reported suffering from low morale.[7] British policy analysts concluded that it is almost as difficult to spend more money effectively in England as it is to control costs in the United States. The basic problem seems to have been that expectations were raised higher than the government could meet.

The election of a conservative-led coalition government in 2010 brought about a plan to institute another wave of sweeping changes in the NHS. The changes seem to have come as surprise to everyone. The objective was to distance politicians from involvement in health care delivery arrangements with the aim of reducing costs. That was to be accomplished by eliminating the Primary Care Trusts and replacing them with GP consortia. At the same time, the GPs were to be given far more authority and funds to negotiate for services to be delivered by hospitals and the specialists employed by hospitals. Hospitals were encouraged to separate from the NHS and become independent non-profit organizations. The public may not have been fully aware of what this would mean. The GPs were divided because they did not believe that they had the administrative background to take on this kind of responsibility and risk. Others in the system pointed out that administrative costs would increase rather than decrease, using the high administrative costs of competition in the United States to make the point. However, the for-profit insurance giants in the United States stepped in, offering to help the Brits with the challenge. So, how well do you expect that to turn out?

Germany

In 2008, Germany was spending $3,737 per person for health care services. The men were living to 76.7 and the women were living to 82.

The German health care system is the oldest national health care system in Europe. It was introduced in 1871 by the government under Otto Von Bismarck (in one part of Germany, Prussia), who reasoned that if the government was thought to be meeting the needs of workers as the country went through industrialization, workers would be less likely to support radical political movements, and his government would stay in control. The current system took shape in 1883 with the passage of the Sickness Insurance Act and applied to all of Germany. The law required all workers below a certain income level to join existing mutual benefit societies, which had established branches that dealt with health care, called sickness funds. The law also required both employees and employers to contribute to the (insurance) premium.

Mutual benefit societies created by guilds and, in some cases, villages to cover the costs of such catastrophes as funerals, lost income resulting from a temporary injury, and permanent disability had been in existence for the last two or three hundred years. People set up these funds to meet the needs they thought were most pressing at the time. Coverage for health care was a secondary consideration until much later because the effectiveness of health care was limited and, what there was, was not costly. By the time that the Sickness Insurance Act was passed, 18,942 sickness funds were already in existence covering 4.7 million people.[8]

The 1883 law gave the funds the authority to establish and operate health clinics. This meant that they were in a position to hire doctors and other staff members. Because the sickness funds were small and run by persons who did not necessarily have the skill to manage large sums of money, doctors were often not paid as promised. They responded by going out on strike whenever that happened. The system could not be described as stable and working to the satisfaction of all involved.[9] Things became more stable during the decade of the 1930s. Interestingly, while doctors were very dissatisfied with prevailing arrangements, they had little influence in shaping the national health insurance system before this time because they had no professional association to represent their views. Germany's doctors organized themselves into a national association in 1931. (Remember, the American Medical Association came into existence in 1847.)

The German health care system evolved as the society modernized, which affected the organization of the sickness funds as well. The number of funds declined over time as some failed and others merged. Enrollment became mandatory for all employees under a government-set income threshold. By the late 1980s, over 90 percent of the population had joined. The self-employed and those whose income was over the income set by the government for mandatory enrollment in a sickness fund (around $66,000 as of 2008) were permitted to buy private insurance coverage. It is widely believed, and there is some evidence to support the idea, that those who are privately insured spend less time waiting to receive care.[10]

Clearly, the federal government has been closely involved in shaping the health care system from the beginning. The system is governed by two principles—solidarity and "subsidiarity," which were written into law in 1949 and to which parties across the political spectrum subscribe, which means that everyone in the country is covered by health insurance.[11] The government sees its role as overseer of the system but does not run the system. It monitors costs and quality. When hospital costs began to rise more rapidly during the mid-1980s, the government stopped paying hospitals whatever they charged and instead required them to operate within a preset budget negotiated at the beginning of the year. This had a significant stabilizing effect.

Doctors are either office-based or hospital-based. Their practices do not overlap. The hospital-based doctors are salaried. The salary is set according to the doctor's specialty and years of experience. Those rates are determined in negotiations between the sickness funds and local physicians' associations. The office-based doctors are paid on a fee-for-service basis, according to a fee schedule established in negotiations between sickness funds and physicians' groups. The fees are also subject to a cap, which works in response to a very interesting and effective mechanism. Medical expenditures are reviewed on a quarterly basis by a unit created by the local medical society. If the total expenditure on office-based physicians' fees exceeds the projected amount, the fees for all office-based practitioners are reduced. Doctors whose fees are significantly higher than those of their colleagues are likely to come under scrutiny—not by bureaucrats, but by a committee of fellow physicians who have the expertise as well as authority to evaluate the reasons behind the high rate. That tends to keep the lid on medical expenditures.

It is worth noting that the German system underwent considerable change during the decade of the 1990s. In part, this was a response to the sudden rise in health care costs that resulted from unification and the additional funds that had to be spent to reorganize the system of care found in East Germany to match the highly technologically advanced system in West Germany. Germany passed health care reform legislation to promote competition among sickness funds in 1993 and again in 1997. The legislation allowed workers greater choice of plans and instituted mechanisms to compensate for the higher costs incurred in caring for higher risk patients. This was done in order to ensure that chronically ill patients were not only recruited by sickness funds because they came with additional compensation, but were receiving treatment.

The most notable effect of the legislation, which promoted competition, was the rapid decrease in the number of sickness funds. Between 1993 and 2004, the number of funds dropped from 1,221 to fewer than three hundred.[12] Another change that took place around this time was the drop in the number of days Germans stay in the hospital—from 15.3 days in 1990 to 11.4 days in 1997.[13] The latter is due to the increase in the number of procedures being performed on an outpatient basis.

One other thing has caused a fair amount of dissatisfaction and upset over recent years. Germans have been very displeased by the government's efforts to control costs through reduction of access to spa treatments. The Germans are great believers in the value of the baths and massages that spas provide. The government has urged sickness funds to reduce coverage from two weeks to ten days or even less.

In the end, Germany is willing to experiment with competition as long as it does not damage the strengths of the existing system and really upset any of the major stakeholders. Put that way, one can understand why the German health care system is not changing very radically or very fast.

France

In 2008, the French were spending $3,696 per person for health care services. The men were living to 76.7 and the women to 83.7.

Although U.S. policy makers are not interested in debating the strengths and weaknesses of the French system, we may want to understand what it is about the system that is causing the World Health Organization to nominate it as the best health care system in the world. Briefly: Basic health insurance coverage is mandatory and linked to occupation. It is obtained through a person's employer. Both the employer and employee share the cost. Individuals may purchase supplementary insurance on top of the basic plan through employment as well. This allows the person to cover additional costs or copayments for office visits, drugs, hospitalization, and so on. As a result, out-of-pocket costs are very low. Also, exemptions for a variety of reasons, for instance, low income, specific diseases, and certain hospital treatments mean that there is no cost-sharing given those circumstances.

As of 2000, those whose income falls under a certain cutoff are entitled to free insurance coverage. Many of the same people have been eligible for financial assistance since 2005 to enable them to purchase insurance. The result is—everyone in the country is covered by health insurance. However, that does not make France unique, since virtually all highly industrialized countries insure everyone in the country. A major part of the explanation for the WHO's rationale for nominating France as the country with the best health care system is that researchers have determined that it achieves the lowest number of *preventable* deaths in comparison to other highly advanced countries due to its health care arrangements. This is known as the "amenable mortality" measure. As of 2003, France had 67 avoidable deaths per 100,000 while the United States had 110 such deaths per 100,000.[14]

Switzerland

Let's consider why some health policy experts wanted us to believe that the Swiss system would be a good model for the United States to emulate.[15] The men live to 79.9 and the women to 84.6, giving them the second longest life expectancy after Japan. However, that was not presented as the primary reason Americans should be interested in the Swiss system. The basic reason was that, while purchase of health insurance is compulsory, people must buy health insurance policies on an individual basis. There are roughly ninety competing plans from which people may choose. There is large out-of-pocket cost. Around 30 percent of the health care bill is paid by individuals rather than insurance. Furthermore, the Swiss have one of the most expensive systems in the world. Ours is, of course, far more expensive at $7,538 per person, and Norway's is next at $4,826 per person, but Switzerland comes as the third most expensive system at $4,463 per person. However, in 2009 Swiss out-of-pocket costs were 30.5 percent and our out-of-pocket costs were only 12.3 percent according to OECD, and, as we know, Americans are very displeased by how much they pay out-of-pocket. The Swiss system was a non-starter once some other observers heard about that. It should be noted that the Swiss seem to be very satisfied with their health care arrangements. The fact that there is very little poverty in Switzerland may explain why so many Swiss people believe their system works well.

Japan

Since the Japanese have had the longest life expectancy in the world for the past several decades, it is worth considering how much their health care system has to do with it. The men were living to 78.6 and the women to 85.5 in 2000. They were spending far less than other advanced countries at $2,729 per person to achieve the highest life expectancy in the world.

The Japanese instituted health insurance in 1927. The country achieved universal coverage by 1961. The Japanese health system relies on over 5,000 insurance plans to organize payment for health care services. About a quarter of the population is covered by self-funded, employer-based plans, meaning that both employees and employers contribute. The proportions paid by employers and employees are similar but not identical from one employer to another. The plans are closely regulated by the government. Another 30 percent of the population is covered under employer-based plans that are government-managed, and partially government-subsidized. The remainder of the population, which includes the self-employed and pensioners, is covered by a plan operated and subsidized by local governments. These premiums are set on the basis of family income.[16]

Americans find Japanese health care arrangements very different from ours. The differences reflect the fact that Japan built its health care system by grafting Western medical practices onto a system based on the delivery of oriental, basically Chinese, medicine. Many doctors advocate the use of herbal medications as well as pharmaceuticals used in Western medicine. They not only prescribe, but dispense both kinds of medications. To put this into context, oriental medicine favors medications and discourages surgery. So there is a lot of prescribing.

Doctors in private practice are permitted to own and operate inpatient clinics with up to 19 beds, which, by law, can be occupied for up to forty-eight hours. Since such doctors do not have hospital privileges, they compete by buying expensive technology for their clinics. The hospitals, especially those associated with prestigious universities, are generally known to offer superior care; however, they do not work on the basis of appointments. So there is an inconvenience tradeoff in going to a superior university hospital or clinic and waiting versus getting a specific appointment at the local doctor's clinic.

Until recently their hospitals have not been nearly as technologically sophisticated as ours, because the Japanese are not eager to spend money on technology that will not produce a good return on the investment. On the other hand, Japanese patients stay in the hospital far longer than Americans do—during the mid 1990s our average length of stay was 5.1 days while theirs ranged from 15.8 to 29.1 days depending on the hospital. This is explained, in large part, by the fact that the Japanese have not been ready to build nursing homes for extended-stay patients. Remember, this is a far more traditional society than ours, where women have historically stayed home and cared for aging parents and sick relatives. More women are now working, but the health care delivery system has not yet caught up. People have dealt with the change in women's roles by checking in their elderly relatives for an extended stay when the work of caring for the aging relative has gotten too burdensome or when they went on vacation. The upshot of the long length of hospital stay is that other patients must wait to be admitted, even those who need immediate attention.

In the spring of 2000, the government agreed to do something about the problem. It passed legislation funding long-term care for the elderly. However, there are very few nursing homes ready to accept elderly patients and Japanese society is not entirely prepared to institutionalize elderly relatives. The shift in attitude and behavior is expected to move forward slowly, making the transition manageable both socially and financially.

When Americans discover that Japanese patients bring their own soap, night clothes, towels, and other necessities to the hospital, including food prepared by the family, they conclude that Japanese hospitals are not nearly modern enough. That is becoming less typical as more women work. However, private nurses have always been and still are a common feature. Finally, Americans find Japanese hospitals to be dingy and extremely short on privacy. For their part, the Japanese are not dissatisfied with their hospitals, which shows, once again, that understandings about comfort and essential amenities are a matter of cultural expectations and values.

How the Japanese managed to spend $2,729 versus our $7,538 per person in 2008 and still achieve the longest life expectancy of any country deserves a little more attention. One reason they can spend so much less is that they have about one-third less surgery than we do. Part of the explanation for the low surgery rate is that organ replacement is culturally unacceptable and restricted by law. Another reason that explains why the Japanese spend less is that they don't have our social problems. They have very little poverty and far less violence, which requires expensive health services, especially emergency room care.

Are there lessons to be learned from the Japanese? By the way, I won't let you dismiss the differences by saying that it is their diet. Yes, their diet plays a critical role; that cannot be denied. But their diet has not changed very much over the last three or four decades when their life expectancy skyrocketed to the top of the international life expectancy scales. It is also true that they have long led the world in the rate of stomach cancer; they smoke at an incredibly high rate, at least the men do; their cities have been highly polluted in the past and are still very crowded; and they work long hours and take little time off, to name a few things that you might expect to detract from their good health. I leave you to ponder these inconsistencies. If you decide to explore this issue in greater detail I recommend that you consider the answer offered by an increasing number of researchers; they believe that social arrangements across social institutions have more to do with the health status of a country's inhabitants than its health care system, which, as a single social institution, cannot overcome factors linked to ill health associated with the operations of other social institutions in the country (e.g., education or labor market).[17]

WHAT ARE WE TO CONCLUDE ABOUT OTHER COUNTRIES' SYSTEMS?

One thing that seems obvious is that different societies have dealt with their concerns about health care in different ways in part because they started doing so at differing times in history. Once their foundations were in place, people just built on top of those foundations. Retrospectively, we can see that the decade of the 1960s, the mid-1980s, and, most recently, during the years just before and after the turn of the twenty-first century, produced some notable reforms in a number of different countries.

The 1960s signaled a period of post–World War II economic growth and prosperity in most countries. Having had a decade to recover from the war, countries turned their attention to internal, social issues. This is when the United States created Medicare and Medicaid and Canada instituted universal health care coverage. During the 1980s, virtually every industrialized country found itself confronting rising health care costs and became convinced that there was no end to it in sight. This is when U.S. policymakers and health care administrators began telling us that competition was the single best solution to the problem of rising costs. Policy makers in other countries found some of the arrangements developed in the United States worth testing. It is interesting to see how competition looks when other countries embrace it. Somehow it does not look much like it does in this country. By the late 1990s, the United States began focusing on mechanisms (i.e., new data collection measures and software to capture trends) designed to measure quality of care. Policy makers in other countries have taken an interest in these developments as well.[18]

Can we, in turn, learn from the experiences of other countries? Perhaps. You might have noticed in reading this chapter that at least one of the mechanisms we created bears a strong similarity to arrangements European countries have had in place for a very long time. Consider the fact that sickness funds, which grew out of mutual benefit societies, were built on the idea that everyone would contribute the same amount of money to maintain the fund even though they would not necessarily benefit from it during any one year, perhaps not ever. Sounds a little like the basis of the Blue Cross plan, doesn't it? Americans celebrated the founding of BC-BS as a totally new idea invented in the United States.

Americans tend toward xenophobia—we seem to have a strong need to reject what is foreign. Unlike the Europeans and Japanese, who have been importing ideas based on our experiments, we prefer to think that we are better off creating new mechanisms from scratch. And we do keep inventing a steady stream of new mechanisms to apply to health care delivery operations, which we are prepared to reject and discard when they fail to deliver what they promised. Then, we simply go on to innovate some more. Winston Churchill's judgment of American ingenuity may be apropos here. He is said to have observed that Americans can be counted on to make the right decisions—after exhausting every other possible option.

· 9 ·

Health Care Policy—
Making the Right Choices

$\mathcal{M}$y purpose in the preceding chapters was, first, to describe how the United States was operating before the Affordable Care Act was passed and, second, to outline the changes mandated by the law. I have no intention of trying to summarize all that information here because, as I suspect you will be quick to agree, there is too much to summarize; and, because as I have said repeatedly, we cannot make concluding statements about something that is in the process of being implemented. This is a very unsettled time—for those working in the health care sector and those tracking how the changes introduced by the new law are faring.

In concluding our discussion, I will use the first half of this chapter to direct your attention to a number of cases that illustrate the difficulties involved in resolving some very practical problems. In the second half of the chapter, I will turn everything we have been saying upside down by raising a really big question, one for which I have provided you with no preparation, namely, whether in focusing on the health care system we have fully explained what is responsible for the less than ideal health profile of people in this country.

CASE STUDIES

Given that we can only identify and discuss a small number of the long list of issues that are on people's minds, we will consider six cases. The cases are timely but not necessarily representative of the larger list of dilemmas confronting us. The objective of this exercise is to consider policy solutions in light of the three health care system goals—access, quality, and cost containment—to evaluate the impact that the solutions being put forth might have on these goals.

Case Number One: The Financial Consequences of
Containing Medicare Program Costs

As you know, based on the discussions presented in previous chapters, among the most contentious issues facing health sector policy makers and politicians is the challenge of identifying funding sources for existing programs known as entitlement programs, meaning Medicare, Medicaid, and Social Security. These programs are so well established that politicians have been unwilling to touch them in the past. They have generally not been ready to argue for decreasing funding let alone eliminating the programs entirely, that is, until recently. At the same time, politicians and policy makers alike agree that the programs' costs are unsustainable.

Whether any changes are made and whether the changes actually reduce costs remains to be seen. Unless we decide to eliminate the programs, which is unlikely, the country will need to find the money to fund the programs at some level because enrollment continues to rise. So, the question is, where will the money come from? Get ready to delve into a very touchy subject— taxes. Everyone seems to agree that closing loopholes in the tax structure is a good thing. However, that's when agreement ends. Warren Buffet, one of the richest men in the country, keeps reminding everyone that he only pays 18 percent in taxes because of all the tax breaks that are available to him. Some other very rich people wish he would just shut up about that. It seems that the majority of people in the country, that is, both Democrats and Independents if not Republicans, are willing to see the tax breaks the rich received under the George W. Bush administration rescinded. How much difference will that make? Apparently not nearly enough to get the country out of its financial difficulties and pay for everything the government is committed to paying for, particularly the entitlement programs plus defense.

A number of possibilities for raising additional funds are being debated. The following outlines one of those possibilities. You know that we are not taxed on the health insurance benefits we get through our employers. According to some calculations, the loss to the government of treating this benefit as nontaxable was $264 billion in 2009. Consider the pros and cons of suddenly eliminating this exemption and treating the amount employers spend on health benefits as taxable income. To begin with, this would largely affect the middle class whose health care coverage is connected to employment. In other words, the tax is not equitable because those who are not covered by employer-sponsored insurance do not enjoy this tax benefit.

Analysts generally agree that the amount of money employers spend comes out of employees' potential income. If employers did not have this expense, the assumption is that they would raise wages and salaries. Of course, we can't be sure about that. It is also worth remembering that if employers were to stop providing health insurance, employees would suddenly have more freedom. They would be in a position to take their insurance with them if they decided to look for another job, a part-time job, for example, in order to use the time to engage in other valued activities, including starting new businesses. In short, this might result in a boost to the economy.

There are a number of other ways people might be taxed other than imposing taxes on health benefits received through employment, all just as unpopular. Politicians could institute taxes on gains resulting from various "financial instruments" or "loopholes," for example, savings plans that allow for tax-free contributions, such as 401(k) plans; or mortgage interest deductions; or other tax breaks enjoyed by investors such as lower rates for dividends and capital gains, and so on.

There really aren't that many alternatives—either find something to tax or cut program expenditures. If we opt for cutting programs, I predict that it would be hard to find programs to cut that would not have some negative financial implications for other programs, as we discovered when we considered the implications of increasing the age of Medicare eligibility. That brings us back to targeting something to tax.

Cutting program costs clearly addresses the goal of cost containment but risks creating negative consequences in terms of the other two health system goals—quality and access. Clearly, we are entering into territory in which purely rational calculations may not provide a fully satisfying answer. Sometimes value judgments have to be taken into consideration.

Case Number Two: Weighing the Social Benefit of Compensating People for Pain and Suffering Versus the Advantages of Reducing Physician Practice Costs

This case goes back to the medical malpractice discussion in chapter four. As we learned in that chapter, California started a trend some years ago that has spread to other states. California set a limit or cap on noneconomic damage awards in malpractice suits. Persons who institute malpractice suits are awarded funds that cover the cost of the treatment, costs of future health care, and costs of lost wages into the future. What is capped is the award for "pain and suffering." In California the cap is set at $250,000. Since then, six other states set caps in most cases on noneconomic damages but in one state on total damages. The caps are now being challenged in the courts.

Why would California set a cap in the first place? The basic reason is that malpractice settlements have an impact on malpractice insurance premium rates, in other words how much doctors pay for malpractice insurance. Once California put the cap in place, the malpractice insurance rate stabilized and did not rise as much as it did in many other states. You may ask why the rest of us should worry about how much doctors have to pay for their malpractice insurance. Well, if the rate is high enough, then doctors seem to think it is a good idea to enter into practice in other states, those that have lower rates. Won't there be enough doctors to pick up the slack? In big cities, it is not a problem. In less populated areas it has been a serious problem. For example, in some regions of the country there are no physicians willing to do obstetrical care, that is, deliver babies. Physicians in small towns just can't charge enough to cover their malpractice costs.

Let's consider the arguments for malpractice caps, pro and con, that the two sides in this debate say they will be presenting in court. The lawyers who have launched the suit say that the threat of malpractice makes doctors more careful and that, in turn, ensures high-quality care. Doctors say that they are doing a lot of unnecessary testing in order to protect themselves from potential lawsuits. They are not doing the tests for the sake of quality. The fact that they do so many unnecessary tests increases the cost of care unnecessarily. Which health system goal should be the priority here? What do you think? Is malpractice a reasonable way to achieve high-quality care even if it ends up costing a lot?

Of course, we don't have to reinvent the wheel. We might want to ask if anyone else is doing a better job of dealing with this issue. If we consider how malpractice works in other countries, we find that there is often a board that determines whether the malpractice suit is legitimate before it is allowed to move forward. There is no such thing as a package settlement covering all pending cases without investigating each individual case. Sweden, for example, uses two separate boards to settle cases. One board determines what the financial settlement should be based on the particular circumstances in the case regardless of whether the doctor can be faulted or not. There is no separate amount set aside for pain and suffering. The other board investigates whether the doctor is at fault or whether the poor outcome was the result of factors out of the doctor's control. This board has the authority to institute sanctions that affect the doctor, the hospital, and any others who might be involved.

Then there is the case of one state that does not wish to have this activity publicized, and the arrangements it has in place to deal with infant mortality. The state employs staff charged with tracking infant mortality by region throughout the state. Every infant death is reviewed. In cases where the cause of death was clearly unavoidable, the death is entered as a statistic and things end there. In instances where the death might have been avoided, a team of physicians and other staff members contacts the hospital where the death occurred and announces that a training session will have to be scheduled. The training session does not charge anyone with making errors. Its purpose is to offer the latest techniques, research, and other information on difficult deliveries. There is no reference to malpractice. The fact that the state infant mortality team did a training session is treated as a matter of routine rather than something that warrants public attention. The rationale is that doctors and other staff will be less reluctant to ask questions and will be more open to absorbing valuable new information if they know that their privacy is protected. The family may or may not initiate a lawsuit, but the fact of the training session is not considered admissible as evidence in court.

So what do you think? Are other countries and this particular state addressing the problem of quality of care in a way that makes sense to you? Or do you think that the threat of a malpractice suit is a better way to ensure quality of care? What about access and cost containment? If we went the route taken in the two examples discussed above, who would be most likely to object? Would patients be hurt if more states decided to pursue malpractice reform by instituting a cap on "pain and suffering" awards?

Case Number Three: Do Patents Encourage Researchers to be Innovative or Do They Restrict Access to Care?

The first human tissue patents in this country were issued to Myriad Genetics for two genes linked to breast cancer some time ago. The company charges $3,000 for the test that determines whether the woman has inherited one or both of the genes that put her at greater risk of breast cancer. No alternative tests have been developed because of the patents. A district court in New York invalidated the patents in March of 2010, stating the patenting of natural phenomena is barred by existing laws. The company argued that the DNA the company has isolated is a chemical not found in nature; therefore it should be exempt from the laws that bar patenting natural phenomena. The company took the case to the appellate court. That case has not yet been heard at this writing. Observers expect the case to go to the Supreme Court regardless of the decision the appellate court reaches. The issue is becoming more pressing as more patents are sought and awarded. Patents now cover about 20 percent of the genome.

A number of organizations opposed to patenting presented *amicus* (friend of the court) briefs in support of the case against patenting. They argued that control over the genes is preventing researchers from improving tests and patients from pursuing second opinions. They argued that genes are certainly a product of nature, just like gold, which cannot be patented.

On the other side are lawyers who practice patent law. They contended that researchers need patents to obtain funding to do research, which they can get if they can assure investors that there will be sufficient return on the investment.

Here, we see cost containment and access in direct opposition and the possibility of risk to future research, which relates to quality. What do you think? Is it reasonable to patent elements of the human genome or should the patents be invalidated?

Case Number Four: How Much Would Information about Doctors' Reimbursement from Medicare Help Stem the Tide of Medicare Fraud?

Senators Chuck Grassley and Ron Wyden introduced a measure during the 2011 congressional session aimed at overriding a law that has been in existence for the last three decades prohibiting the release of Medicare billing data. The senators' proposal involves publishing online the amount of Medicare reimbursement doctors receive. The intent is to curb fraud by identifying those who are overcharging. The AMA is campaigning against this proposal because it considers this to be an unwarranted invasion of privacy. The AMA has no objection to the procedures Medicare is using currently to identify physicians whose charges are excessive, which leads to investigation of those doctors' treatment practices. The AMA notes that all physicians are expected to use an electronic medical record filing system in the near future, which should make finding outliers much easier without violating physicians' privacy.

Medicare fraud is a major problem. It is not clear that physician billing practices are responsible for the majority of the fraud or costs of fraud. To illustrate, in the autumn of 2010, a fraudulent operation was identified when the bad guys submitted a claim under an obstetrical Medicare code requesting funding for delivery of a baby—for someone on Medicare? It turns out that a gang of foreign mobsters in California had somehow gotten hold of Medicare numbers of New York state residents. It was only when they made a dumb mistake that they got caught.

The most recent fraud scheme, which is not defrauding the Medicare program directly, has con men telling Medicare enrollees that they will have to obtain a new Medicare card, which the con men say they will furnish but they need the person's social security number. That allows them to get into bank accounts and empty them. No one seems to know how to institute controls that would detect fraud connected to Medicare on a consistent basis.

The question before the Congress is whether releasing doctors' billing records, which may or may not achieve cost containment, is justified or whether the privacy of doctor's income information is a more important consideration. In concentrating on cost containment, we are clearly moving further away from access and quality, but the matter of curbing fraud seems to be high on the political agenda. Can you see any other ways to curb fraud that affects Medicare and other programs?

Case Number Five: Dietary Supplements—Supply, Demand, and Regulation

Because dietary supplements are not drugs, they are not regulated by the Federal Drug Administration (FDA), the government agency that monitors drugs in this country. Dietary supplement manufacturers are not required to list the active ingredients, nor are they required to provide a list of possible adverse effects. There are no standards for the amount of active ingredient involved or the purity of the ingredients. Tainted products tend to be identified only after a certain number of people experience complications. Products may be banned if enough people sicken or die from ingesting them. Then the problem is preventing the products from entering the country or being sold over the Internet, which involves other government agencies. At the other extreme, the supplements may have no active ingredients—they may consist of nothing but refined sugar. The topic began receiving attention in the late 1990s, when prominent members of the medical establishment raised the alarm. The concern was that people were taking the supplements along with prescription drugs and not telling their physicians. People were suffering adverse effects due to overdosing. The Bureau of Consumer Protection got involved in 2003. It charged several companies with fraud in claiming that ephedra, the weight loss supplement, would have no side effects. It was ultimately banned because so many people got sick and some died after using it. The same year, Senators Orrin Hatch and Joseph Biden said they would present a bill aimed at preventing the sale of steroids, used for bodybuilding; however, the bill did not get very far. *Consumer Reports* began issuing annual reports on the detrimental side effects of dietary supplements the following year. The issue has gotten attention in waves since then. It hit the news again in August of 2011, when the *New York Times* reported that a recent study found that "Americans spent $28.1 billion dollars last year, up from $21.3 billion five years ago" on dietary supplements.[1]

The question here is a classic one. Do you believe that the government should step in to institute more controls, which would presumably reduce the public's access to supplements, probably increase costs, without necessarily guaranteeing increased quality or assurance of effectiveness? Or do you believe that the market is doing a good enough job of balancing quality, access, and cost and that the government should stay out of the picture? Does the fact that so many people are buying these products, given that the expenditures are in the $28 billion range, play a role in your answer to this question?

Case Number Six: Allocating a Scarce Commodity—What Values Should Apply?

Scarcity is central to the process of organ replacement surgery. This is not a new problem. It just seems to erupt periodically, as it has recently. What do you think? Should young people who are healthier and have years of life ahead of them go to the front of the line when an organ, say, a kidney, becomes available? Or should those who have been on the waiting list the longest and have suffered all that time waiting for a kidney get the first available one that matches? Years ago, the teams that matched those needing a transplant with available organs met and made the decision based on who was most deserving as well as most needy. Then issues like whether the potential recipient was married and had dependent children entered into the equation. When even that was not enough to make the determination, other factors were considered, for example, whether the person was worthy based on previous history—whether he or she had ever abused drugs, was contributing to society through a worthwhile job—as you can see this produced a very slippery slope. Making judgments about who is more deserving is not something that can be done without a lot of bias. The question regarding whether time spent waiting for an organ replacement should be considered has not been completely settled and continues to be debated. What do you think is the right answer?

In this case we have moved away from the three health care system goals to focus on ethics. There are many issues under this heading that we will not be taking up. But think about it—there is the question of whether doctors should assist people who wish to end their lives because they cannot bear to suffer any more. One state, Oregon, permits this; the others do not. What do you think? Then there is the question of whether doctors should be doing artificial insemination, which produces a large number of embryos, for anyone who can afford it, and let parents select which embryo they wish to implant? Does their reason for doing this matter? If they want a genetic match to a sick older child who would benefit from a blood transfusion when the embryo becomes old enough to be a donor—is that a good enough reason? Is the sex of the child a good reason for making the selection? What about all the other embryos? Is it okay to use all those embryonic cells for research purposes or should they be destroyed? We could go on to identify more cases, but what we have discussed so far should give you plenty to think about.

ARE THERE OTHER CONSIDERATIONS THAT WE HAVE NOT ADDRESSED?

Now that we have considered a number of cases dealing with unresolved issues out of the long list of possible cases, let me ask you this. Do you think that we might not have given sufficient attention to some other variables that probably have a fair amount of impact on people's health status in previous chapters? Indeed, I am suggesting that the question that we have not addressed is how much does access to health care matter when you step back and consider who is healthy and why they are healthy? Maybe health status and life expectancy depend on something other than what the health care system can deliver. I realize that it is a little late to raise that issue now, but let's give it some thought before we part.

The simple answer is that we can say without reservation that access to health care goods and services does make a significant difference to a person's health status. Obviously, variation in quality simply magnifies the difference. And cost is major factor in whether people have access or not. Is that it? If people have access to high-quality health care services that they can afford, will that ensure that those people are healthier and live longer? Let's look at the evidence.

The Institute of Medicine brought together a panel of experts to examine the evidence regarding the question of whether health care matters in 2002.[2] The panel concluded that about 18,000 Americans die prematurely every year because they do not have access to health care services. A 2008 update calculates that the number of deaths comes closer to 22,000.[3] Another extensive review of the literature carried out in 2002, under the auspices of the Kaiser Commission on Medicaid and the Uninsured, found that having health insurance reduces mortality rates by 10 to 15 percent; that not having it means that people are more likely to be diagnosed at a later stage of illness; not having it means that they are more likely to be hospitalized for an avoidable condition; and, beyond that, the commission determined that poor health affects educational attainment, which reduces earnings potential by 10 to 30 percent.[4]

We know that people are more likely to take the medications they were prescribed when cost sharing is reduced or eliminated.[5] We know that when people do not seek out preventive care services and/or delay care, that increases costs because health problems become more serious if they are not treated in the early stages. Similar insights were responsible for the health maintenance legislation way back in 1974. But we seem to forget such things.

I probably do not need to point out that the emphasis here is on health care coverage, that is, insurance, rather than health care per se. That is due to the fact that researchers can calculate the presence or absence of health insurance. Utilization of health care services is much more complicated because people may choose not to seek health care services for reasons other than not having insurance or the money to pay for care. People might have an asymptomatic problem like high blood pressure; they might not want to face up to a problem they do know they have; they might fear the treatment; they might be afraid that they will lose their jobs if they take time away from work for treatment, and so on.

Returning to the question that I raised a moment ago, does having access to health care explain all or almost all of the variation in life expectancy and illness rates, that is, mortality and morbidity? For example, is it possible that people's behavior is the primary factor that explains differences in health status, including bad habits such as smoking, eating junk food, not exercising? Or maybe it's our genes, which we can't do anything about, genes that make some of us more susceptible to obesity, cancer, diabetes, or heart disease.

Our views regarding how big a role these factors play has an impact on how we decide to apportion the country's health care dollars. There is no question that we are allocating the largest amount of money to addressing health problems after they occur. Some people argue that we should be putting greater emphasis on prevention of health problems before they occur. That would mean increasing funding for programs to help people avoid addiction to cigarettes, alcohol, drugs; teaching people the risks of using tanning salons; teaching them how to improve their diets, and so on. Of course, if we are convinced that health is mostly a matter of genetic inheritance, then we should be shifting a greater proportion of public resources to research on genetic mapping, screening, and pharmaceutical breakthroughs designed to alter our genetic predispositions.

Then there are all those sociocultural factors that seem to be so closely related to poor health, such as poverty, discrimination, and inadequate education with the impact that has on ability to earn a good living. There is little disagreement about the fact that people who have less education have fewer prospects for getting a good job, a nice house in a safe neighborhood, and all the other things that characterize a comfortable middle-class lifestyle. But why do they also exhibit the highest levels of morbidity and mortality? Is it because they don't know that smoking, bad diet, and addiction to drugs or alcohol is bad for their health? Hardly likely. They know what is bad for their health and do it anyway. It is this phenomenon that requires an explanation.

Researchers who have been working on identifying factors that are linked to health status and longevity have come up with an answer. It is more complicated than it looks at first glance. The explanation can be summed up as having less money—not being impoverished, just having less money than other people have to buy things. What things? All those things that are so aggressively advertised and that one sees other people buying—things like running shoes, electronic gadgets, and clothes with designer labels displayed so prominently. What is it, you may ask, about being able to afford all this stuff that is linked to health status? This is where things get really interesting.

A fascinating branch of the research in this field indicates that the answer to the question of how much money is enough is—it's relative. In other words, it is not one's actual income and certainly not need for all that stuff that is being advertised. It is one's purchasing power relative to everyone else's purchasing power in the society in which one lives that is relevant. What people in other societies are buying does not seem to matter nearly as much as what people in one's own society can buy. How does one define one's society? It is made up of neighbors, coworkers, and, of course, all those really, really wealthy celebrities whose personal lives we hear so much about that they seem almost like relatives.

Remember the discussion on economic inequality in chapter one where we learned that a small proportion of Americans are becoming extremely rich while many more are becoming poorer? Americans may not be aware of those statistics. What they do know is that they cannot buy the things that others can buy. That realization is exactly what makes the people who cannot afford to buy all the stuff that is being advertised feel left out of the mainstream of society. What is relevant to this discussion is that these people also experience the highest rates of morbidity and mortality.

If the perception that one does not have enough money to buy the kinds of things others can buy has important effects on health, what is the logical health policy response? According to Richard Wilkinson and Kate Pickett, whose work we have been referring to throughout the book, access to health care services is essential. However, they say that it is the sense of social and economic inequality we are seeing in this country that is central to explaining our high mortality and morbidity rates compared to populations in other advanced countries.[6] It is the degree of inequality that people are experiencing that is stressing them out and making them feel that someone needs to be blamed for the dissatisfaction they are feeling about their lives. Social inequality is what is causing so many people to feel they are living in a society which is not allowing them to participate fully, making them feel that they cannot count on one another and must protect themselves from being taken advantage of by others including the government they no longer trust; feeling that their voices don't matter, so why bother voting; and, in the end, why bother trying to live in a way that will bring about longer life expectancy? Why not take drugs? Why not engage in violence against those who have so much more?

So what is the solution? According to Richard Wilkinson and Kate Pickett, the answer is obvious. They say that reducing socioeconomic inequality would increase the level of trust we have in our social institutions and each other, which would, in turn, reduce the degree of divisiveness we see in this country. Reducing socioeconomic inequality would go a long way in helping us agree to make social changes that would benefit all of us. Perhaps it would even dissuade some people from investing so much energy in working to overturn measures that benefit all of us and devoting themselves to working to institute measures aimed at protecting the advantages accruing to those who are already in the top income bracket.

That is, of course, a very tall order. Maybe we could start with some smaller steps. Maybe the suggestion made by Rashi Fein, the medical economist whose observations we have mentioned in earlier chapters, might be a place to start. In his view, educating people would help them understand that

> insurance that provides protection against life-altering expenditures has great value, and that [if] it has been necessary to use it one hasn't "wasted one's money." Perhaps the overriding lesson is that we need to invest more resources in voter education.[7]

In short, extending health insurance to everyone in the country and helping them understand its value is an excellent first step in helping us all move toward a shared sense of values.

Drew Altman, president and CEO of the Kaiser Family Foundation, whose research reports we have relied on throughout the book, makes the case for educating the public more firmly. He makes his sense of frustration about Americans' understandings about health care reform explicit in suggesting, only partially in jest, that we should forget teaching students English and math and instead teach them how laws are made and the impact that major pieces of legislation, particularly the Affordable Health Act, can have.[8]

As I hope that you are firmly convinced by now, the ACA is certain to have a profound effect on all Americans. At the most basic level, it can be expected to produce an improvement in the health status of so many who have not had access to health care services prior to this time. At another, far less concrete level, it might bring about a greater sense of inclusiveness. Given the record exhibited by all other advanced societies, we can expect the increased sense of inclusiveness to be reflected in a range of other indicators of well-being, from such disparate measures as the rate of teenage pregnancy and violent crime, and numbers of people who are incarcerated, to the level of innovation and creativity represented by the number of patents the country can claim. But these are topics for a whole new book. I have written on this subject in my book *Unequal Health*.[9]

In conclusion, I hope you come away from *Our Unsystematic Health Care System* with a stronger sense of the health care system in the United States, why it looks the way it does, the role that public opinion plays in shaping our system, and the scope of the changes under way. At times, the study of these topics seems to raise more questions than answers, but by approaching the discussion from an informed perspective, you will be equipped to help shape the health of our country.

Notes

CHAPTER 1

1. "Life Expectancy at Birth and at 65 Years of Age, by Sex: Organisation for Economic Co-operation and Development (OECD) Countries, Selected Years 1980–2007," *Health, United States, 2010: With Special Feature on Death and Dying* (Hyattsville, MD: National Center for Health Statistics, 2011), table 21 (online at http://www.cdc.gov/nchs/data/hus/2010/021.pdf).

2. "Infant Mortality Rates and International Rankings: Organisation for Economic Co-operation and Development (OECD) Countries, Selected Years 1960–2007," *Health, United States, 2010: With Special Feature on Death and Dying* (Hyattsville, MD: National Center for Health Statistics, 2011) table 20 (online at http://www.cdc.gov/nchs/data/hus/2010/020.pdf).

3. Richard Wilkinson and Kate Pickett, *The Spirit Level: Why Greater Equality Makes Societies Stronger* (New York: Bloomsbury Press, 2009), PowerPoint slides, slide 31.

4. Richard G. Wilkinson, *Unhealthy Societies: The Afflictions of Inequality* (London: Routledge, 1996).

CHAPTER 2

1. Thomas Piketty and Emmanuel Saez, "Income Inequality in the United States, 1913–1998," *Quarterly Journal of Economics* 118 (February 2003): 1–39. (Tables and figures updated to 2008 on the Emmanuel Saez web site, July 2010, http://elsa.berkeley.edu/~saez/.)

2. Robert Reich, "Foreword," in Richard Wilkinson and Kate Pickett, *The Spirit Level: Why Greater Equality Makes Societies Stronger* (New York: Bloomsbury Press, 2010), vi.

3. Michael Norton and Dan Ariely, "Building a Better America—One Wealth Quintile at a Time," forthcoming in *Perspectives on Psychological Science* (Spring 2011).

4. Bureau of Labor Statistics, *The Consumer Price Index: Concepts and Content over the Years* (Washington, DC: U.S. Department of Labor, 1978).

5. Robert J. Blendon and John M. Benson, "Americans' Views on Health Policy: A Fifty-Year Historical Perspective," *Health Affairs* 20 (March 2001): 33–46.

6. U.S. Department of Health and Human Services, "The 2011 HHS Poverty Guidelines" (online at http://aspe.hhs.gov/poverty/11poverty.shtml).

7. Blendon and Benson, "Americans' Views," 34.

8. Blendon and Benson, "Americans' Views," 34–35.

9. Rashi Fein, *Learning Lessons: Medicine, Economics, and Public Policy* (New Brunswick, NJ: Transaction Publishers, 2010).

10. Blendon and Benson, "Americans' Views," 43.

11. Kevin Sack and Marjorie Connelly, "In Poll, Wide Support for Government-Run Health," *New York Times* (June 20, 2009).

12. For an insider's assessment of the change in tactics used by the health insurance industry regarding the health care reform debate prior to passage of health care reform legislation see: Wendell Potter, *Deadly Spin: An Insurance Company Insider Speaks Out on How Corporate PR Is Killing Health Care and Deceiving Americans* (New York: Bloomsbury Press, 2010).

13. Mollyann Brodie, Drew Altman, Claudia Deane, Sasha Buscho, and Elizabeth Hamel, "Liking the Pieces, Not the Package: Contradictions in Public Opinion During Health Reform," *Health Affairs* 29 (June 2010): 1125–1130.

14. Brodie et al., "Liking the Pieces," 1126.

15. Husna Haq, "Why Americans Oppose the Health Care Reform Bill," *The Christian Science Monitor* (March 19, 2010) (online at https://www.csmonitor.com/USA); Drew Altman, "Pulling It Together: Forget Math and Science, Teach Civics (Or Why We Need to Bring Back 'Schoolhouse Rock')," Henry J. Kaiser Family Foundation (February 24, 2011).

16. Institute of Medicine, *Insuring America's Health: Principles and Recommendations* (Washington, DC: National Academies Press, 2004), 155.

17. Tara Sussman, Robert J. Blendon, and Andrea Louise Campbell, "Will Americans Support the Individual Mandate?" *Health Affairs* 28 (May 2009): w501–w509.

18. U.S. Department of Health and Human Services. Centers for Medicare and Medicaid Services, National Health Expenditure Data, NHE Fact Sheet (online at https://NationalHealthExpendData/25_NHE-Fact_Sheet.asp).

19. NHE Fact Sheet.

20. "National Health Expenditures, Average Annual Percentage Change, and Percent Distribution by Type of Expenditure: United States, Selected Years 1960–2008," *Health, United States, 2010: With Special Feature on Death and Dying* (Hyattsville, MD: National Center for Health Statistics, 2011), table 125 (online at http://www.cdc.gov/nchs/data/hus/2010/125.pdf).

CHAPTER 3

1. E. H. L. Corwin, *The American Hospital* (New York: Commonwealth Fund, 1946).

2. Rosemary Stevens, *In Sickness and in Wealth* (New York: Basic Books, 1989).

3. "Hospital Service in the United States," *Journal of the American Medical Association* 90 (April 3, 1928): 1009.

4. "National Health Expenditures, Average Annual Percentage Change, and Percent Distribution by Type of Expenditure: United States, Selected Years 1960–2008," *Health, United States, 2010: With Special Feature on Death and Dying* (Hyattsville, MD: National Center for Health Statistics, 2011), table 125 (online at http://www.cdc.gov/nchs/data/hus/2010/125.pdf). "The National Bill: The Most Expensive Conditions by Payer, 2008," Statistical Brief #107, Healthcare Cost and Utilization Project (Rockville, MD: Agency for Healthcare Research and Quality, March 2011) (online at www.hcup-us.ahrq.gov/reports/statbriefs/sb107.pdf).

5. "Discharges, Days of Care and Average Length of Stay in Nonfederal Short-Stay Hospitals by Selected Characteristics: United States, Selected Years 1980–2007," *Health, United States, 2010: With Special Feature on Death and Dying* (Hyattsville, MD: National Center for Health Statistics, 2011), table 99 (online at http://www.cdc.gov/nchs/data/hus/2010/099.pdf).

6. The Combined Budget Reconciliation Act of 1985 (COBRA), which prohibits hospitals receiving Medicare funds from transferring unstable patients and women in active labor until they are stabilized, went into effect on August 1, 1986.

7. Eugene Declercq and Diana Simmes, "The Politics of 'Drive-Through Deliveries': Putting Early Postpartum Discharge on the Legislative Agenda," *The Milbank Quarterly* 75, no. 2 (1997): 175–202.

8. "Uninsured Hospital Stays, 2008," Statistical Brief #108, Healthcare Cost and Utilization Project (Rockville, MD: Agency for Healthcare Research and Quality, April 2011) (online at www.hcup-us.ahrq.gov/reports/statbriefs/sb108.pdf).

9. David Classen, Roger Resar, Frances Griffin, Frank Federico, Terri Frankel, Nancy Kimmel, John C. Whittington, Allan Frankel, Andrew Seger, and Brent C. James, "'Global Trigger Tool' Shows that Adverse Events in Hospitals May Be Ten Times Greater than Previously Measured," *Health Affairs* 30 (April 2011): 581–89.

10. Jill Van Den Bos, Karan Rustagi, Travis Gray, Michael Halford, Eva Ziemkiewicz, and Jonathan Shreve, "The $17.1 Billion Problem: The Annual Cost of Measurable Medical Errors," *Health Affairs* 30 (April 2011): 596–603.

11. See: April issue of *Health Affairs* entitled: Gaps in Health Care Quality Persist.

12. John A. Romley, Anupam B. Jena, and Dana P. Goldman, "Hospital Spending and Inpatient Mortality: Evidence from California, An Observational Study," *Annals of Internal Medicine* 154 (February 2011): 160–67.

13. "CMS's Special Focus Facility Methodology Should Better Target the Most Poorly Performing Homes Which Tend to be Chain Affiliated and For-Profit," GAO-09-689 (Washington, DC: United States Government Accountability Office, August 2009).

CHAPTER 4

1. Howard Becker, Blanche Geer, Everett C. Hughes, and Anselm L. Strauss, *Boys in White: Student Culture in Medical School* (Chicago: University of Chicago Press, 1961), 419–33; Robert K. Merton, George G. Reader, and Patricia L. Kendall, eds., *The Student-Physician: Introductory Studies in the Sociology of Medical Education* (Cambridge, MA: Harvard University Press, 1957), 295–96.

2. Committee on Quality of Health Care in America, Institute of Medicine, Linda T. Kohn, Janet H. Corrigan, Molla S. Donaldson, eds., *To Err Is Human: Building a Safer Health System* (Washington, DC: National Academy Press, 1999), 26.

3. Michelle M. Mello, Amitabh Chandra, Atul A. Gawande and David M. Studdert, "National Costs of the Medical Liability System," *Health Affairs* 29 (September 2010): 1569–77.

4. Tanya Albert, "Malpractice Plaintiffs' Wins, Awards Up slightly," *American Medical News* (April 19, 2004): 8.

5. "Special Update on Medical Liability Crisis," U.S. Department of Health and Human Services, Office of the Assistant Secretary for Planning and Evaluation (September 25, 2002) (online at http://aspe.hhs.gov/daltcp/reports/mlupd1.htm).

6. Alicia Gallegos, "Medical Liability Premiums Steady, But Big Extremes Remain," *American Medical News* (January 17, 2011): 14–15.

7. J. William Thomas, Erika C. Ziller, and Deborah A. Thayer, "Low Costs of Defensive Medicine, Small Savings from Tort Reform," *Health Affairs* 29 (September 2010): 1578–84.

8. Paul Starr, *The Social Transformation of American Medicine* (New York: Basic Books, 1982), 112–23.

9. Abraham Flexner, *Medical Education in the United States and Canada* (New York: The Carnegie Foundation for the Advancement of Teaching, 1910).

10. Grace Budrys, *When Doctors Join Unions* (Ithaca, NY: Cornell University Press, 1997).

11. Linda Aiken, Sean Clarke, Robyn Cheung, Douglas Sloane, and Jeffrey Silber, "Educational Levels of Hospital Nurses and Surgical Patient Mortality," *Journal of the American Medical Association* 290 (September 24, 2003): 1617–23; Linda McGillis Hall, Diane Doran, G. Ross Baker, George Pink, Souraya Sidani, Linda O'Brien-Pallas, and Gail Donner, "Nurse Staffing Models as Predictors of Patient Outcomes," *Medical Care* 41 (September 2003): 1096–1109; Julie Sochalski, "Is More Better?: The Relationship Between Nurse Staffing and the Quality of Nursing Care in Hospitals," *Medical Care* 42 (February 2004): II-67–II-73; Jack Needleman, Peter Buerhaus, Soeren Nattke, Maureen Stewart, and Katya Zelevinsky, "Nurse-Staffing Levels and the Quality of

Care in Hospitals," *New England Journal of Medicine* 346 (May 30, 2002): 1715–22; Kevin Grumbach, Michael Ash, Jean Ann Seago, and Janet Coffman, "Measuring Shortages of Hospital Nurses: How Do You Know a Hospital with a Nursing Shortage When You See One?" *Medical Care Research and Review* 58 (December 2001): 387–403.

12. Charles Fiegl, "Skepticism Greets Medicare ACO Shared Savings Program," *American Medical News* (April 18, 2011): 1–2.

13. Carolyne Krupa, "Psychologists Seek Prescribing Rights In 6 States," *American Medical News* (March 7, 2011): 1, 4 (online at http://www.ama-assn.org/amed news/2011/03/07/prl20307.htm).

CHAPTER 5

1. Sylvia A. Law, *Blue Cross: What Went Wrong?* (New Haven, CT: Yale University Press, 1974), 6–12.

2. Rosemary Stevens, *In Sickness and In Wealth* (New York: Basic Books, 1989), 259.

3. Bruce Japsen, "Illinois Blues Balk at Go-Public Stampede," *Chicago Tribune.* (June 10, 1999), 1, 4.

4. Gail Jensen, Michael Morrisey, Shannon Gaffney, and Derek Liston, "The New Dominance of Managed Care: Insurance Trends in the 1990s," *Health Affairs* 16 (January/February 1997): 125–36.

5. "Persons Enrolled in Health Maintenance Organizations (HMOs) by Geographic Region and State: United States, Selected Years 1980–2002" (Washington, DC: U.S. Department of Health and Human Services, Public Health Service, 2003), table 150.

6. Mark Hall and Christopher Conover, "The Impact of Blue Cross Conversions on Accessibility, Affordability, and the Public Interest," *Milbank Quarterly* 81 (2003): 509–42.

7. "Medicare Enrollees and Expenditures and Percent Distribution, According to Type of Service: United States and Other Areas, Selected Years 1970–2001," *Health, United States, 2003, with Chartbook on Trends in the Health of Americans*, U.S. Department of Health and Human Services (Hyattsville, MD: National Center for Health Statistics, 2003), table 134.

8. Maurissa Kanter and MacKenzie Lucas, "U.S. Health Care Cost Rate Increases Reach Highest Levels in Five Years According to New Data from Hewitt Associates" www.hewitt.com (September 27, 2010).

9. Robert Kazel, "Union Seeks to Limit Aetna Execs' Pay," *American Medical News* (April 12, 2004): 20.

10. Emily Berry, "Profits Keep Rolling in for Big Insurers Despite Reform," *American Medical News* (February 21, 2011): 32–33.

11. "Private Health Insurance Coverage Obtained through the Workplace among Persons under 65 Years of Age, by Selected Characteristics: United States, Selected Years 1984–2009." *Health, United States, 2010: With Special Feature on Death and Dying*

(Hyattsville, MD: National Center for Health Statistics, 2011), table 136 (online at http://www.cdc.gov/nchs/data/hus/2010/136.pdf).

12. Henry J. Kaiser Family Foundation and Health Research & Educational Trust, "Employer Health Benefits: 2010 Summary of Findings," Survey #8085. n.d. (online at http://ehbs.kff.org/pdf/2010/8086.pdf).

13. "Private Health Insurance Coverage among Persons under 65 Years of Age, by Selected Characteristics: United States, Selected Years 1984–2009," *Health, United States, 2010: With Special Feature on Death and Dying* (Hyattsville, MD: National Center for Health Statistics, 2011), table 135 (online at http://www.cdc.gov/nchs/data/hus/2010/135.pdf).

14. Donna Dubinsky, "Money Won't Buy You Health Insurance," *New York Times* (February 20, 2011): 10.

15. Sara Collins, Michelle Doty, Ruth Robertson, and Tracy Garber, "Help on the Horizon: How the Recession Has Left Millions of Workers Without Health Insurance, and How Health Reform Will Bring Relief—Findings from the Commonwealth Fund Biennial Health Insurance Survey of 2010," publication of The Commonwealth Fund, www.commonwealthfund.org (March 16, 2011).

16. Robert Pear, "Health Care Overhaul Depends on States' Insurance Exchanges," *New York Times* (October 23, 2010): 23.

CHAPTER 6

1. "Medicare: Medicare Advantage Fact Sheet," Henry J. Kaiser Family Foundation and Health Research & Educational Trust (March 2004) (online at http://www.kff.org/medicare/upload/Medicare-Advantage-Fact-Sheet.pdf).

2. Marsha Gold, "Medicare's Private Plans: A Report Card on Medicare Advantage," *Health Affairs* 28 (January/February 2009): w41–w54; Kim Bailey, "Whose Advantage? Billions in Windfall Payments Go to Private Medicare Plans," Families USA Special Report (June 2007): 4 (online at http://www.familiesusa.org/assets/pdfs/medicare-private-plans.pdf).

3. Marsha Gold, Gretchen Jacobson, Anthony Damico, and Tricia Neuman, "Medicare Advantage 2011 Data Spotlight: Plan Availability and Premiums," Henry J. Kaiser Family Foundation (October 2010) (online at http://www.kff.org/medicare/upload/8117.pdf).

4. Robert Pear and Edmund Andrews, "White House Says Congressional Estimate of New Medicare Costs Was Too Low," *New York Times* (February 2, 2004): A14.

5. "Long-term Care: Baby Boom Generation Presents Financing Challenges." Testimony before the Special Committee on Aging, U.S. Senate, Statement of William Scanlon, Director Health Financing and Systems Issues (Washington, DC: United States General Accounting Office, 1998), 4 (online at http://www.gao.gov/archive/1998/he98107t.pdf).

6. "2011 Annual Report of The Boards of Trustees of Federal Hospital Insurance and Federal Supplementary Medical Insurance Trust Funds," Boards of Trustees, Fed-

eral Hospital Insurance and Federal Supplementary Medicare Insurance Trust Funds (May 13, 2011).

7. Lynn Etheredge and Judith Moore, "A New Medicaid Program," *Health Affairs* web exclusive (August 27, 2003) (online at http://content.healthaffairs.org/content/early/2003/08/27/hlthaff.w3.426/suppl/DC1).

8. National Clearinghouse for Long-Term Care Information, U.S. Department of Health and Human Services (online at www.longtermcare.gov).

9. Joel Finkelstein, "Millions Have Health Coverage Gaps—Commonwealth Fund Study," *American Medical News* (December 1, 2003): 10–11.

10. "SCHIP: HHS Continues to Approve Waivers That Are Inconsistent with Program Goals," United States Government Accountability Office, GAO-04-166R (January 5, 2004) (online at http://www.gao.gov/new.items/d04166r.pdf).

11. "Two-Thirds of Medicaid Eligible Children Not Enrolled," National Center for Policy Analysis (September 9, 2010) (online at http://www.ncpa.org/sub/dpd/index.php?Article_ID=19802).

12. "Raising the Age of Medicare Eligibility: A Fresh Look Following Implementation of Health Reform," Henry J. Kaiser Family Foundation Program on Medicare Policy, publication number 8169 (March 29, 2011) (online at http://www.kff.org/medicare/upload/8169.pdf).

CHAPTER 7

1. John Holahan, "Will Health Care Reform Increase the Deficit and National Debt?: Timely Analysis of Immediate Health Policy Issues," Urban Institute, Robert Wood Johnson Foundation (August 2010) (online at http://www.urban.org/UploadedPDF/412182-health-reform-deficit.pdf).

2. Robert Blendon, Drew Altman, Claudia Deane, John Benson, Mollyann Brodie, and Tami Buhr, "Health Care in the 2008 Presidential Primaries," *New England Journal of Medicine* (January 24, 2008): 414–22.

3. Jacob Hacker and Paul Pierson, *Winner-Take-All Politics: How Washington Made the Rich Richer—And Turned Its Back on the Middle Class* (New York: Simon and Schuster, 2010), 109.

4. Kaiser Family Foundation, "Kaiser Public Opinion Spotlight: Health Care and Elections" (updated April 2008). (online at http://www.kff.org/spotlight)

5. CNN Opinion Research Corporation, "CNN/Opinion Research Poll" (December 16–20, 2009) (online at http://politicalticker.blogs.cnn.com/2009/12/21/cnnopinion-research-poll-december-16-20-2009/).

6. Kaiser Family Foundation, "Kaiser Tracking Poll. Public Opinion on Health Care Issues" (May 21, 2010) Kaiser poll #8075 (online at http://www.kff.org/kaiserpolls/trackingpoll.cfm).

7. Drew Altman, "Pulling it Together: Health Reform's Six-Month Checkup," Kaiser Family Foundation (September 27, 2010) (online at http://www.kff.org/pullingittogether/Health-reforms-six-month-checkup.cfm).

8. "Americans Remain Divided Over Health Reform with an Uptick in Public Opposition as GOP Ramped Up Repeal Campaign," Kaiser Family Foundation (January 25, 2011) (online at http://www.kff.org/kaiserpolls/posr012511nr.cfm).

9. Drew Altman, "Pulling It Together: Forget Math and Science, Teach Civics (Or Why We Need to Bring Back 'Schoolhouse Rock')" Henry J. Kaiser Family Foundation (February 24, 2011).

10. Richard S. Foster, "Estimated Financial Effects of the 'Patient Protection and Affordable Care Act,' As Amended," Centers for Medicare and Medicaid, Office of the Actuary (April 22, 2010) (online at http://www.cms.gov/ActuarialStudies/Downloads/PPACA_2010-04-22.pdf).

11. Richard G.Wilkinson, *Unhealthy Societies: The Afflictions of Inequality* (London: Routledge, 1996); Ichiro Kawachi, Richard Wilkinson, and Bruce Kennedy, *The Society and Health Population Reader, Vol. 1: Income Inequality and Health* (New York: The New Press, 1999); Michael Marmot and Richard G. Wilkinson, *Social Determinants of Health* (Oxford, UK: Oxford University Press, 1999); Richard Wilkinson and Kate Pickett, *The Spirit Level: Why Greater Equality Makes Societies Stronger* (New York: Bloomsbury Press, 2009).

12. Kenneth Arrow, "Uncertainty and the Welfare Economics of Medical Care," *American Economic Review* 53 (December 1963): 941–73.

13. Marcia Angell, *The Truth About the Drug Companies: How They Deceive Us and What to Do About It* (New York: Random House, 2004); Shannon Brownlee, *Overtreated: Why Too Much Medicine Is Making Us Sicker and Poorer* (New York: Bloomsbury, 2007); Jerome Kassirer, *On the Take: How Medicine's Complicity with Big Business Can Endanger Your Health* (New York: Oxford University Press, 2005); Melody Peterson, *Our Daily Meds: How the Pharmaceutical Companies Transformed Themselves into Slick Marketing Machines and Hooked the Nation on Prescription Drugs* (New York: Farrar, Straus and Giroux, 2008).

14. Rashi Fein, *Learning Lessons: Medicine, Economics, and Public Policy* (New Brunswick, NJ: Transaction Publishers, 2010).

15. The Physicians' Working Group for Single-Payer National Health Insurance, "Proposal of the Physicians' Working Group for Single-Payer National Health Insurance," *Journal of the American Medical Association* 290 (August 13, 2003): 798–805.

16. Physicians' Working Group, "Proposal," 798.

17. David Himmelstein, Deborah Thorne, and Steffie Woolhandler, "Medical Bankruptcy in Massachusetts: Has Health Reform Made a Difference?" *The American Journal of Medicine* 124 (March 2011): 224–28.

18. Kevin Sack and Marjorie Connelly, "In Poll, Wide Support for Government-Run Health," *New York Times* (June 21, 2009).

19. Steffie Woolhandler and David Himmelstein, "Paying for National Health Insurance—and Not Getting It," *Health Affairs* 21 (July 2002): 88–98.

20. Wilhelmine Miller, Elizabeth Richardson Vigdor, and Willard Manning, "Covering the Uninsured: What Is It Worth?" *Health Affairs* web exclusive (March 31, 2004): w4-157–167.

21. Wilkinson and Pickett, *The Spirit Level*, 40–62, 211.

22. Wilkinson and Pickett, *The Spirit Level*, 235.

23. Kaiser Family Foundation, "Health Care Spending in the United States and Selected OECD Countries," Henry J. Kaiser Family Foundation (April 2011) (online at http://www.kff.org/insurance/snapshot/OECD042111.cfm).

CHAPTER 8

1. Robert Blendon, Robert Leitman, Ian Morrison, and Karen Donelan, "DataWatch: Satisfaction with Health Systems in Ten Nations," *Health Affairs* 9 (Summer 1990): 185–92.

2. Julia Abelson, Matthew Mendelsohn, John Lavis, Steven Morgan, Pierre-Gerlier Forest, and Marilyn Swinton, "Canadians Confront Health Care Reform," *Health Affairs* 23 (May/June, 2004): 186–93.

3. Carolyn Hughes Tuohy, "Dynamics of a Changing Health Sphere: The United States, Britain, and Canada," *Health Affairs* 18 (May/June, 1999): 129.

4. Odin Anderson, *Health Care: Can There Be Equity? The United States, Sweden, and England* (New York: Wiley-Interscience, 1972).

5. Joseph White, *Competing Solutions: American Health Care Proposals and International Experience* (Washington, DC: The Brookings Institution, 1995), 121.

6. Rudolf Klein, "Britain's National Health Service Revisited," *The New England Journal of Medicine* 350 (February 26, 2004): 937–42; Peter Smith and Nick York, "Quality Incentives: The Case of U.K. General Practitioners," *Health Affairs* 23 (May/June, 2004): 112–18; Simon Stevens, "Reform Strategies for the English NHS," *Health Affairs* 23 (May/June, 2004): 37–44.

7. Klein, "Britain's National Health Service," 937.

8. John Iglehart, "Germany's Health Care System (First of Two Parts)," *The New England Journal of Medicine* 324 (February 14, 1991): 503–8.

9. Deborah Stone, *The Limits of Professional Power: National Health Care in the Federal Republic of Germany* (Chicago: University of Chicago Press, 1980).

10. Katherine Leith, Astrid Knott, Alexander Mayer, and Jorg Westermann, "Germany," in *Comparative Health Systems: Global Perspectives*, edited by James Johnson and Carleen Stoskopf (Sudbury, MA: Jones and Bartlett Publishers, 2010), 160.

11. Leith et al., "Germany," 158.

12. Leith et al., "Germany," 156.

13. Lawrence Brown and Volker Amelung, "'Manacled Competition': Market Reforms in German Health Care," *Health Affairs* 18 (May/June, 1999): 88.

14. Ellen Nolte and C. Martin McKee, "Measuring the Health of Nations: Updating an Earlier Analysis," *Health Affairs* 27 (January/February 2008): 58–71.

15. Organisation for Economic Co-operation and Development (OECD), OECD Health Data 2011, Frequently Requested Data (online at http://oecd.org/document/16/0,3343,en_2649_34631_2085200_1_1_1_1,00.html).

16. Naoki Ikegami and John Creighton Campbell, "Health Care Reform in Japan: The Virtues of Muddling Through," *Health Affairs* 18 (May/June, 1999): 56–75; John Iglehart, "Japan's Medical Care System," *The New England Journal of Medicine*

319 (September 22, 1988): 807–12; Naoki Ikegami and John Creighton Campbell, "Japan's Health Care System: Containing Costs and Attempting Reform," *Health Affairs* 23 (May/June, 2004): 26–36; M. G. Marmot and George Davey Smith, "Why Are the Japanese Living Longer?" *British Medical Journal* 299 (December 23–30, 1989): 1547–51.

17. Richard Wilkinson and Kate Pickett, *The Spirit Level: Why Greater Equality Makes Societies Stronger* (New York: Bloomsbury Press, 2009).

18. Peter Hussey, Gerard Anderson, Robin Osborn, Colin Feek, Vivienne McLaughlin, John Millar, and Arnold Epstein, "How Does the Quality of Care Compare in Five Countries?" *Health Affairs* 23 (May/June 2004): 89–99.

CHAPTER 9

1. Natasha Singer, "Here's to Your Health, So They Claim," *New York Times, Sunday Business* (August 28, 2011): 1, 6.

2. Institute of Medicine, *Care Without Coverage: Too Little, Too Late* (Washington, DC: National Academy Press, 2002).

3. Stan Dorn, "Uninsured and Dying Because of It: Updating the Institute of Medicine Analysis on the Impact of Uninsurance on Mortality," Urban Institute (January 2008) (online at http://www.urban.org/publications/411588.html).

4. Jack Hadley, "Sicker and Poorer: The Consequences of Being Uninsured," prepared for the Kaiser Commission on Medicaid and the Uninsured, Henry J. Kaiser Family Foundation, 2002 (online at http://www.kff.org/uninsured/upload/Full-Report .pdf); Kaiser Commission on Medicaid and the Uninsured, "The Uninsured, A Primer: Key Facts about Americans Without Health Insurance" (The Henry J. Kaiser Family Foundation, 2006) (online at http://www.kff.org/uninsured/upload/7451.pdf).

5. See November 2010 issue of *Health Affairs*.

6. Richard Wilkinson and Kate Pickett, *The Spirit Level: Why Greater Equality Makes Societies Stronger* (New York: Bloomsbury Press, 2009).

7. Rashi Fein, *Learning Lessons: Medicine, Economics, and Public Policy* (New Brunswick, NJ: Transaction Publishers, 2010), 171.

8. Drew Altman, "Pulling it Together: Forget Math and Science, Teach Civics (Or Why We Need to Bring Back 'Schoolhouse Rock')," Henry J. Kaiser Family Foundation (February 24, 2011).

9. Grace Budrys, *Unequal Health: How Inequality Contributes to Health or Illness* (Lanham, MD: Rowman & Littlefield Publishers, 2010).

Index

access, 5, 26, 105, 141, 145

Accountable Care Organizations (ACOs), 44–45, 66

Affordable Care Act (ACA), 1–2, 14, 17, 18–19, 24, 26, 44–45, 65–67, 69, 83, 90, 94, 103, 105, 108–109, 111, 152

Agency for Healthcare Research and Quality (AHRQ), 39

allopathic medicine, 48–49

alternative medicine, 48

American Association of Medical Colleges, 56, 61

American College of Physicians, 67

American College of Surgeons, 32–34

American Hospital Association, 33–34

American Medical Association (AMA), 34, 55, 59, 67, 74–75, 79, 133, 146

American Nurses Association, 61

Arrow, Kenneth, 115

Australia, 121–23

Blue Cross-Blue Shield (BC-BS), 36, 70–73, 83, 139

Bureau of Labor Statistics (BLS), 21, 47, 59

Canada, 121, 122–27

capitation, 75, 129

caveat emptor, 115–19

Census Bureau, 23

Centers for Medicare and Medicaid Services (CMS), 27, 41, 45, 58, 66, 93–94, 106, 111

CHIP. *See* State Child Health Insurance Program

Civil War, 16–17

Clinton era, 22–23

Combined Budget Reconciliation Act of 1986 (COBRA), 83

Commonwealth Fund, 83

competition, 9, 127

computerized axial tomography scanner (CT), 4, 38, 123, 126

Congressional Budget Office (CBO), 107, 111

consumer-driven health care, 78

consumer price index (CPI), 21

cost containment, 5, 41, 105–106, 141, 145

cost-shifting, 38, 71, 112

"death panels," 109

Department of Health and Human Services (HHS), 31, 42–43, 66, 93, 99

Diagnostic Related Groups (DRGs), 37–38

dietary supplements, 147–48

disproportionate share hospitals (DSH),
    39, 44, 107

economic inequality, 8, 16–17, 151
electronic medical records, 54–55
emergency medical technicians, 63
employer mandates, 25–26, 85–86
England. *See* United Kingdom
entitlement programs, 89

Federal Drug Administration (FDA), 48
Federal Insurance Coverage Act (FICA),
    18, 20
Federal Trade Commission (FTC), 79
Federally Qualified Health Centers
    (FQHCAs), 42
fee-for-service, 14, 70, 75, 128, 134
Flexner, Abraham, 55
Flexner Report, 56
France, 121–22, 135

Germany, 121, 132–34
Government Accountability Office
    (GAO), 78
Great Depression, 18, 20, 26, 34, 70
Great Recession, 15, 39, 94
gross domestic product (GDP), 27, 122,
    130

Health Benefit Exchanges, 84–87
health care costs, 21
health insurance, 10, 13–14, 22
premiums, 70–73, 75, 81
private health insurance, 8, 69; public
    health insurance, 8, 69. *See also*
    Medicaid, Medicare, and State Child
    Health Insurance Program
Health Maintenance Organization
    (HMO), 22, 66–67, 74–80, 116;
    HMO premium, 75
Health Resources and Services
    Administration (HRSA), 42
Health Savings Accounts, 78

health care reform, 20–26, 47, 83,
    85; health care reform employer
    requirements, 85–86
health care reform options, 25
Hill-Burton Act, 34–35
home health care, 43
hospices, 43
hospital administrators, 64
Hospital Quality Alliance, 41
hospitals, 27, 29–46; community, 30–31;
    for-profit, 30–31, 40–41; nonprofit,
    30–31; public, 30; safety net, 39;
    Veterans Administration, 30

indemnity, 72
Independent Payment Advisory Board,
    44, 65, 106
Individual health insurance market,
    81–83, 86
individual mandates, 25–26
inpatient, 38
Institute of Medicine (IOM), 25, 53,
    118, 149
Italy, 121–22

Japan, 3, 121–23, 135–38
Johns Hopkins Medical School, 56
Joint Commission on Accreditation of
    Healthcare Organizations (JACHO),
    34, 36, 93–94

Kaiser Family Foundation, 80, 102, 109,
    111, 149, 152
Kaiser Permanente, 70, 74–75
Kennedy-Johnson era, 21, 23

length of stay, 37–38, 40
life expectancy, 2–3, 19
long-term care facilities, 29, 42, 137. *See
    also* nursing homes

magnetic resonance imaging (MRI), 38,
    123, 126

malpractice, 38, 52, 127, 143–45; and tort reform, 53
managed care, 76
managed competition, 77
market. *See* competition
Medicaid, 21–22, 26, 36–37, 65, 75, 83, 89, 97–102, 106, 112–13, 118, 138; beneficiaries, 97–98; enrollees, 97–98; means testing, 89, 100; spend down, 99
medical bankruptcy, 117–18
medical education, 55–57
medical-loss ratio, 78, 85, 103
"medical home," 66
medical profession, 48–59
medical specialization, 49–52
Medicare, 1, 21–22, 24, 26, 36–37, 40–41, 43–44, 65, 75, 89–97, 101–102, 106–108, 113–14, 118, 138, 142–43, 146; Part A, 90, 95; Part B, 90, 95; Part C, 90, 92, 95, 107. *See also* Medicare Advantage; Part D, 90, 92–93, 95–96, 110. *See also* Medicare Prescription Drug, Improvement, and Modernization Act
Medicare solvency, 19
Medicare Prescription Drug, Improvement, and Modernization Act, 90
medigap insurance, 91–112
moral hazard, 115

National Bureau of Economic Research, 15
National Center for Health Statistics, 2
National Health Service Corps (NHSC), 42
Netherlands, 121–22
never events, 44
Nixon era, 22–23, 74–75
nurses, 47, 59–62; advanced practice nurses, 62, 67
nursing homes, 27, 43

occupancy rates, 38
ophthalmology, 49–50
Organization for Economic Co-operation and Development (OECD), 122–23
osteopaths, 48–52
outpatient, 38, 42

patients, 145–46
Patient-Centered Outcome Research Institute, 65
Patient Protection and Affordable Care Act. *See* Affordable Care Act
Peer Review Organizations (PROs), 9
pharmaceutical companies, 116n13
physicians' assistants, 63
physicians' earnings, 58; reimbursement from Medicare, 146
podiatrists, 64
point of service plans, 78
positron emission tomography (PET), 38
poverty, 17, 22, 85, 100
poverty line, 21, 23
pre-paid care, 74
prescription drugs, 27
primary care practitioners (PCPs), 52, 77
private sector, 8
public opinion polls, 4–5, 24–25, 105–20
public sector, 8

quality, 5, 32, 37, 41, 105–106, 133, 141, 145–46

Reich, Robert, 16
Resource Based Relative Value Scale (RBRVS), 58
risk rating, 72

Saez, Emmanuel, 16
SCHIP. *See* State Child Health Insurance Program

Single-payer plan, 25, 117–18, 125–27
social institution, 10–11, 128, 138
Social Security Act, 18, 20, 26, 89, 97
Social Security Administration, 19
Social Security Trust Fund, 18–20, 90
socialized medicine, 13–75, 128
specialty hospitals, 44–45
State Child Health Insurance Program
    (SCHIP or CHIP), 26
Sweden, 3, 144
Switzerland, 123, 135–36

Tea Party, 26, 108, 113
technicians, 63

therapists, 62
Truman era, 20, 23
trust in government, 23, 25

United Kingdom, 6, 13, 121–22, 124,
    128–32
U.S. Department of Justice, 79
U.S. Office of Personnel Management,
    84

Wilkinson, Richard and Kate Pickett,
    119, 151
World War II, 15, 20, 34–35, 50, 72,
    128, 138

About the Author

Grace Budrys is professor of sociology at DePaul University. She chaired the committee charged with creating the Masters of Public Health Program a few years ago and now teaches in that program. Before completing her doctorate at the University of Chicago, she worked in various health care organizations, including a university teaching hospital, a nonprofit dedicated to overcoming a leading cause of mortality, and a hospital consulting firm. Her research and teaching interests evolved from a focus on health organizations and occupations, resulting in two earlier books, *Planning for the Nation's Health* and *When Doctors Join Unions*. More recently she has been focusing her attention on health disparities, which she addresses in the book *Unequal Health*, now in its second edition. Her continuing interest in how Americans get their health care and how those arrangements continue to change is captured in each of the revisions of *Our Unsystematic Health Care System*.

CPSIA information can be obtained at www.ICGtesting.com
Printed in the USA
BVOW031649061111

275349BV00002B/3/P